Gestational Trophoblastic Disease

Bhagyalaxmi Nayak • Uma Singh
Editors

Gestational Trophoblastic Disease

Benign to Malignant

Springer

Editors
Bhagyalaxmi Nayak
Associate Professor
Department of Gynaecologic Oncology
Acharya Harihar Post Graduate Institute of Cancer
Cuttack
India

Uma Singh
Professor & Head
Department of Obstetrics and Gynecology
King George's Medical University
Lucknow
India

ISBN 978-981-33-4877-6 ISBN 978-981-33-4878-3 (eBook)
https://doi.org/10.1007/978-981-33-4878-3

This Springer imprint is published by the registered company Springer Nature Singapore Pte Ltd.
The registered company address is: 152 Beach Road, #21-01/04 Gateway East, Singapore 189721, Singapore

Foreword

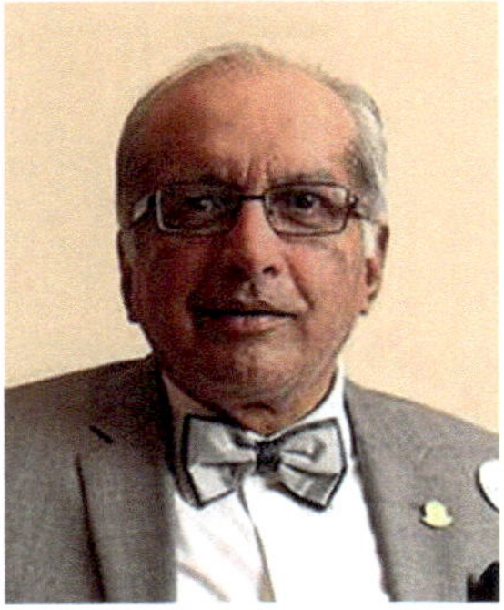

Medical science is evolving everyday, and to keep up with rapidly changing knowledge about any subject, it is mandatory to bring out a book which comprehensively covers all the aspects.

Gestational trophoblastic disease, a condition found fairly commonly in this part of the world, has often not been adequately covered in standard textbooks. This book is focused on the whole spectrum of benign to malignant form of this disease in a comprehensive manner. It contains updated information written in a simple yet lucid manner and hence would serve as a valuable text and reference book for practicing gynecologic oncologists, gynecologists, and postgraduate students and fellows.

It gives me pleasure to write this foreword for this concise book, and I convey my best wishes to the editors and contributing authors of the book.

Dr C. N. Purandare
President FIGO 2015-18, President FOGSI 2009,
Emeritus Dean Indian College of Obstetrics & Gynaecology
Mumbai, India

Consultant: O&G, St. Elizabeth Hospital, BSES and Saifee Hospital
Mumbai, India

Foreword

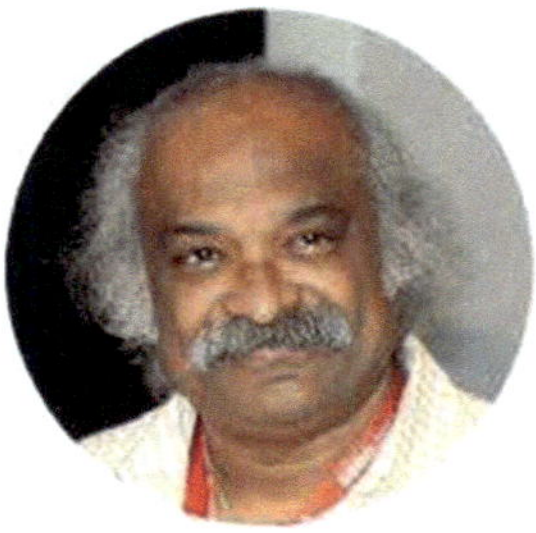

With advancing knowledge in medical science in various fields and technological breakthrough, conceptual transformation, and changing modalities of diagnosis and therapy of a particular disease like gestational trophoblastic disease, it is absolutely essential to bring out a book that comprehensively covers all the aspects from basic to advance.

Gestational trophoblastic disease (GTD), God's first cancer and man's first cure, is not uncommon in a country like India. Moreover, there is a lot of confusion and lack of consensus starting from the classification to diagnosis and treatment modalities. Aiming in these aspects, this book is focused and dedicated in covering all the spectrum from benign to malignant in a lucid manner in different chapters. The galaxy of authors and their contribution in various sections of this book will definitely help the practicing gynecologists, oncologists, and postgraduate students in understanding this disease with clarity, and I am sure this would serve as a valuable text and indispensable reference book for the readers.

I thank all the contributing authors and editor of this book and convey my best wishes. It gives me pleasure to write this foreword for this concise Bible.

Dr P. C. Mahapatra
President FOGSI 2011, Ex Prof. & HOD, SCB Medical College
Cuttack, India

Consultant & IVF Specialist, Prachi Institute of Mother & Child Health
Cuttack, India

Contents

About the Editors

Dr. Bhagyalaxmi Nayak M D, FICOG, PhD is faculty in the postgraduate department of gynecologic oncology in Regional Cancer Center, Cuttack, India. She is fellow of the Indian College of Obstetrics and Gynecology. She has many publications and has delivered many lectures at national and international conferences. She was the vice president of the Association of Gynecologic Oncologists of India and chairperson of the Oncology Committee of FOGSI. She was the executive publisher of *Indian Journal of Gynecologic Oncology* and presently is an Assistant Editor of the same. She has been awarded the YUVA FOGSI Oration and the Usha Saraiya Oration in gynecologic oncology. She is the principal investigator of project on the role of bacterial vaginosis in cervical cancer funded by the Department of Science & Technology. She is a PhD guide to students at Ravenshaw University.

Professor Uma Singh MD, FICOG is Dean, King George Medical University and professor in the department of Obstetrics and Gynecology at King George Medical College, Lucknow. She has several publications in national and international journals and has been the guide for many theses and PhD projects. She is a reviewer for *International Journal of Applied and Basic Medical Research, Indian Journal of Gynecologic Oncology, and Journal of Obstetrics and Gynecology of India*. She is member of South Asia Expert Group for Prevention of Cancer Cervix. She also has a fellowship in Advanced Course in Medical Education.

Gestational Trophoblastic Disease: An Overview

1

S. K. Giri

Gestational Trophoblastic Disease (GTD) includes a spectrum of interrelated pregnancy-associated diseases where abnormal growth disturbances of human trophoblast occur manifesting a wide range of biologic behaviour. More than 80% of GTD cases are benign in nature, though all have potentiality for malignant transformation of any magnitude. As a neoplastic disease, GTD is derived from foetal tissue, but exclusively invades maternal tissue. Production of large quantities of hCG is a hallmark. Spontaneous regression is possible—less in Choriocarcinoma. Because of haematogenous spread—it mimics good number of other pathologic conditions. This is the first disseminated solid tumour to be cured by Chemotherapy. Though commonly five clinico-pathological forms of GTD are recognised, a sixth entity "Atypical Placental Site Nodule" (APSN) has recently been included.

1. Hydatidiform mole (HM)
   (a) Complete Hydatidiform Mole (CHM)—(Fig. 1.1)
   (b) Partial Hydatidiform Mole (PHM)
2. Invasive Mole (IM)
3. Gestational Choriocarcinoma (CCA)
4. Placental Site Trophoblastic Tumour (PSTT)
5. Epithelioid Trophoblastic Tumour (ETT)

The entire above are grouped under GTD in a broad term. CHM and PHM are termed as premalignant/potentially malignant GTD. Malignant form of GTD is termed as Gestational Trophoblastic Neoplasia (GTN) (otherwise called persistent GTD) and this term is reserved for those requiring CT. GTN encompasses, CCA, IM, PSTT and ETT. The persistent elevation and plateauing of hCG without any

S. K. Giri (✉)
Department of Gynaecologic Oncology, A.H. Post Graduate Institute of Cancer, Cuttack, India

B. Nayak, U. Singh (eds.), *Gestational Trophoblastic Disease*,
https://doi.org/10.1007/978-981-33-4878-3_1

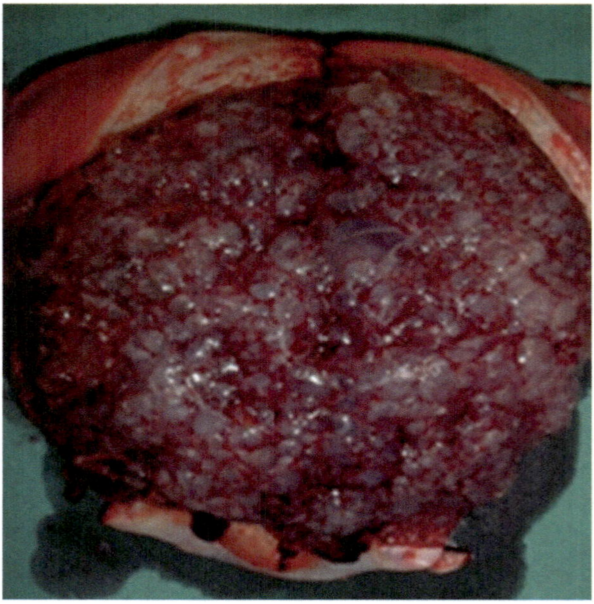

Fig. 1.1 Cut open uterus with complete mole in situ

other clinical or radiological evidence of the disease is also a GTN and is not essential to make a histological verification for a diagnosis of GTN. CCA, PSTT and ETT are diagnosed only by histopathological examination of the tissue, and PSTT and ETT are classified separately. It is observed that about 15–20% of CHM and 0.5–5% of PHM on follow-up after evacuation, develop to GTN and require chemotherapy [1, 2]. Choriocarcinoma of ovary and testes is grouped under **Non-gestational** Trophoblastic disease.

1.1 Aetiology of GTD

About 80% of CHM are diploid. This results from duplication of the haploid single sperm after fertilisation of the ovum in which maternal chromosomes are lost during meiosis, resulting in 46xx androgenic conceptus. Fertilisation of this ovum devoid of maternal genetic material by two sperms may give rise to XX or XY conceptus, which happens in about 20% of cases. In such situation, there is failure of embryogenesis and the trophoblastic tissue undergoes hyperplasia with hydropic changes and formation of vesicles.

PHM is the product of fertilisation error. An apparently normal ovum containing 23X haploid set of chromosomes is fertilised by two spermatozoa, commonly one with 23X and other with 23Y paternal haploid set of chromosomes, resulting in 69XXY.PHM is thus diandric triploid.

PSTT is a rare type of GTD that arises in the uterus at the site where the placenta was implanted. These tumours are locally invasive and penetrate the muscle layer of the uterus and usually do not spread to other parts of the body. PSTT is composed mainly of implantation type of intermediate cytotrophoblastic cells. It produces hPL more than hCG.

ETT is a rarest of Trophoblastic tomours composed of chorionic type of intermediate trophoblast. Its biological behaviour appears similar to PSTT.

1.2 Diagnosis and Management

The diagnosis of HM is nearly always made by strong clinical suspicion of the disease and confirmed by ultrasound. Colour Doppler USG is an additional armamentarium in diagnosing and predicting the outcome of HM. Once diagnosis is made, serum β-hCG estimation is done to have baseline data, which facilitates post-treatment follow-up and further management. Further investigations like X-Ray chest, USG, CT scan/MRI of chest, brain and abdomen and pelvis, though not routinely required, and may be done as situation demands.

1.2.1 Treatment

Suction & Evacuation is the treatment of choice, ideally under ultrasound guidance with a large bore canula. Judicious use of oxytocics before, during and after evacuation to prevent uterine atony is now advocated, though one should keep in mind the risk and danger of embolism. After the uterus is empty gentle sharp curettage may be performed to remove residual tissue. The specimen obtained from suction and sharp curettage should separately be submitted for histopathologic examination. Check curette done only if incomplete evacuation. Rh immunoglobulin should be given to Rh negative mother unless there is absolute confirmed evidence of CHM. Hysterectomy may be done when indicated with preservation of ovaries.

1.3 Follow-Up After Evacuation

- Weekly β-hCG estimation to undetectable level.
- After normalisation, further weekly estimation β-hCG is done twice.
- Subsequently, estimation is done every month up to 6 months.
- After that β-hCG measurement should be done every 3 months for 6 months, to establish an apparent cure or rule out early relapse.

Patients, whose β-hCG falls within the 56th day of evacuation, fall into short "follow-up group" and further pregnancy is allowed after 6 months. When β-hCG fall takes more than 56 days, these patients fall into "long follow-up group" and follow-up is required in them up to 2 years with β-hCG estimation monthly for 1 year, than 3 monthly for second year.

Contraception in terms of barrier is advised. However, OCP can be advocated after the β-hCG level reaches normal.

1.3.1 Prophylactic Chemotherapy

About 20% of patients of HM will require chemotherapy because of rise or plateau of β-hCG during the course of follow-up. Hence prophylactic chemotherapy is no longer advocated to all or some patients of HM, as this exposes 80% of the patient to unnecessary chemotherapy and its inherent toxicity. Moreover, prophylactic should only be offered to patients who cannot be followed up or risk of developing postmolar GTN is high [3, 4]. But the irony is that, prophylactic chemotherapy does not prevent follow-up or development to GTN. The authors of Cochrane Database of Systematic Reviews 2017 on prophylactic chemotherapy, observed no consensus regarding dosage, regimen and number of cycles. Moreover, in case, development of GTN after prophylactic chemotherapy, the patients needed more cycles of chemotherapy or alternative agents, as they become resistant to usual chemotherapy. Hence the authors are not in favour of recommending its use in clinical practice [4].

1.3.2 Gestational Trophoblastic Neoplasia

Gestational Trophoblastic Neoplasia (GTN) is a rare malignant disease, which can be cured even in advanced stages. About 50% GTNs follow a molar pregnancy, the rest occur after any pregnancy events.

1.3.3 Criteria for Diagnosis of Postmolar GTN

The diagnosis of post-molar GTN is made as per criteria laid down by FIGO 2018 [5].

- Four or more plateaued measurements over a period of 3 weeks or more, i.e. days 1, 7, 14, 21.
- Rise in hCG for three consecutive weekly measurements over at least a period of 2 weeks or more; days 1, 7, and 14.
- Histological diagnosis of Choriocarcinoma.

1.4 Hammond's South-Eastern Trophoblastic Disease Centre Clinical Classification of GTD [6]

- No metastatic disease—no evidence of disease outside the uterus.
- Metastatic disease—any disease outside uterus.
  - Good prognostic metastatic disease.

    Short duration (last preg. <4 months).

Low pretreatment serum hCG titre (<40,000 IU/L or urinary hCG < 100,000 IU/24 hours).
No metastatic to brain or liver.
No antecedent term pregnancy.
No significant prior chemotherapy.

– Poor prognosis metastatic disease.
Long duration (last preg. > 4 months).
High pretreatment serum hCG titre >40,000 IU/L or Urinary hCG > 100,000 IU/24 hours).
Brain or liver metastases.
Significant prior chemotherapy.
Antecedent term pregnancy.

1.5 Management of GTN

Management depends on risk factors as defined. Non-metastatic and low-risk metastatic GTN Risk score ≤ 6 are usually treated with single-agent chemotherapy like Methotrexate and Actinomycin D in different dose schedules. Five FU and oral Etoposide do give excellent results. Patients with metastatic high-risk GTN (risk score ≥ 7) will require multi-agent chemotherapy like EMACO.

Role of second curettage—GOG [7] conducted a study of 64 patients on the second curettage in low risk and non-metastatic GTN regardless of hCG levels and intrauterine disease and observed that chemotherapy can be avoided in 47% of such cases with a score of ≤ 4 after second curettage, whereas no benefit was observed in patients with a score of 5–6. On the contrary, an RCT [8] conducted from October 2011 through February 2019 on 89 patients concluded that, second curettage in low-risk GTN has no effect on the number of chemotherapy required, both in control and in study arm. Perhaps more number of studies with meta-analysis of all RCTs accruing more number of patients may resolve this issue of debulking effect of second curettage in future.

In low-risk GTN, at least one course, usually 2–3 courses of CT should be given beyond first negative hCG level. And in high-risk patients requiring multi-agent CT will require 3–4 courses of CT after achieving normal hCG. It is known that more than 10^7 live cells are required to produce detectable hCG.

About 5–15% treated with single-agent CT will require multi-agent CT with or without surgery to achieve complete remission. About 20% with multi-agent CT will become resistant and require other combination CTs like EMA-EP, BEP and other combinations including Taxol and Carboplatin.

A new terminology **"ultra high-risk"** has evolved with a risk score of ≥ 13. It is important to recognise them, as management differs. Early death can be avoided with low dose induction Etoposide and cisplatin [9].

1.6 Follow-Up after Treatment of GTN

1.6.1 Recommendation for Follow Up Is

1.6.1.1 In Low-Risk GTN

1. Weekly hCG assessment until normal for three consecutive weeks.
2. Monthly assessment of hCG till 12 consecutive normal values.

1.6.1.2 In High-Risk GTN

1. Weekly estimation of β-hCG until normal for three consecutive weeks.
2. Monthly estimation of β-hCG for 24 consecutive normal values.

Prolonged follow-up justified in high-risk GTN because higher chance of late recurrence. Though pregnancy is allowed after 1 year of normalisation of hCG, few guidelines advocate follow-up at least up to 5 years [10].

1.6.2 Role of Surgery in GTD

1. S&E primary treatment.
2. Hysterectomy—in excessive bleeding, in tumour-resistant Foci, in perforating mole, PSTT, ETT, patients with high risk of developing GTN, >40 years completed child bearing.
3. Thoracotomy—to remove chemo-resistant foci.
4. To control acute bleeding and to excise resistant focus hepatic resection may be required.
5. To provide acute decompression and to control bleeding, craniotomy may be required.
6. Biopsy from any site is avoided—it may cause fatal haemorrhage.

1.6.3 Quiescent GTD

1. Elevated real hCG—50–100 mIU/ml—encountered after HM or incidentally.
2. Patients have no clinical/imagiological disease.
3. No response to CT/Surgery.
4. After several weeks to years, hCG re-elevated in 20% of cases when the disease is evident.
5. When the disease is evident after re-elevation of hCG, it responds to chemotherapy.

1.6.4 Phantom hCG

Sometimes hCG continues to remain positive at a low level without any evidence of trophoblastic disease or any pregnancy associated event. When the positive hCG value is due to heterophilic antibody, or otherwise a false positive value, is considered as phantom hCG. Presence of phantom hCG is confirmed by repeating the serum hCG assay in dilution, where the value does not decline in proportion to dilution and urinary hCG remains negative.

1.7 WHO Scoring System Based on Prognostic Factors [5]

Risk factors	0	1	2	4
Age in years	<40	>40	–	–
Antecedent pregnancy	Mole	Abortion	Term	–
Interval from index pregnancy in months	<4	4–6	7–12	12
Pre-treatment hCG Milli Iu/ML	$<10^3$	$>10^3$ to 10^4	$>10^4$ to 10^5	$>10^5$
Largest tumour size including uterus	–	3–4 cm	≥5 cm	–
Site of metastases including uterus	Lung	Spleen kidney	GI tract	Brain, liver
Number of metastases identified	–	1–4	5–8	>8
Previous failed chemotherapy	–	–	Single drug	Two or more drugs

Patients with a risk score of 0–6 are grouped under low-risk category and managed with single-agent chemotherapy. A score of seven or greater is categorised as high-risk disease, and patients of high-risk disease are treated with combination chemotherapy.

It is observed that WHO risk score 5–6 and diagnosis of Choriocarcinoma are associated with resistance to single-agent chemotherapy, though they stratified under the low-risk category. These patients may need thoughtful consideration for early initiation of multi-agent chemotherapy [5].

1.7.1 Pregnancy After Mole

Both HM and GTN can expect fare chance of pregnancy after complete treatment. However, these patients should be informed of the increased risk of having a molar gestation in subsequent conception. During first trimester, pelvic USG should be done to confirm normal gestational development. Moreover, after abortion or delivery, following previous molar event, the conceptus or placenta should be subjected to histopathology examination in women who have received chemotherapy to rule out GTD. β-hCG estimation should be done in such patients after 6 weeks postpartum to rule out GTN development. There is no need for hCG estimation and subjecting conceptus and placenta for pathologic evaluation, after normal pregnancy following molar event managed without chemotherapy [11].

1.7.2 To Summarise

Almost all patients with GTD can be cured with modern protocol of management with good fertility outcome. With the present available clinical features and investigations, it is not yet much possible to predict those HM that are likely to progress to

GTN and those GTNs that will become resistant to single-agent chemotherapy enabling early appropriate treatment. Novel biomarkers need to be identified to identify and predict such eventualities.

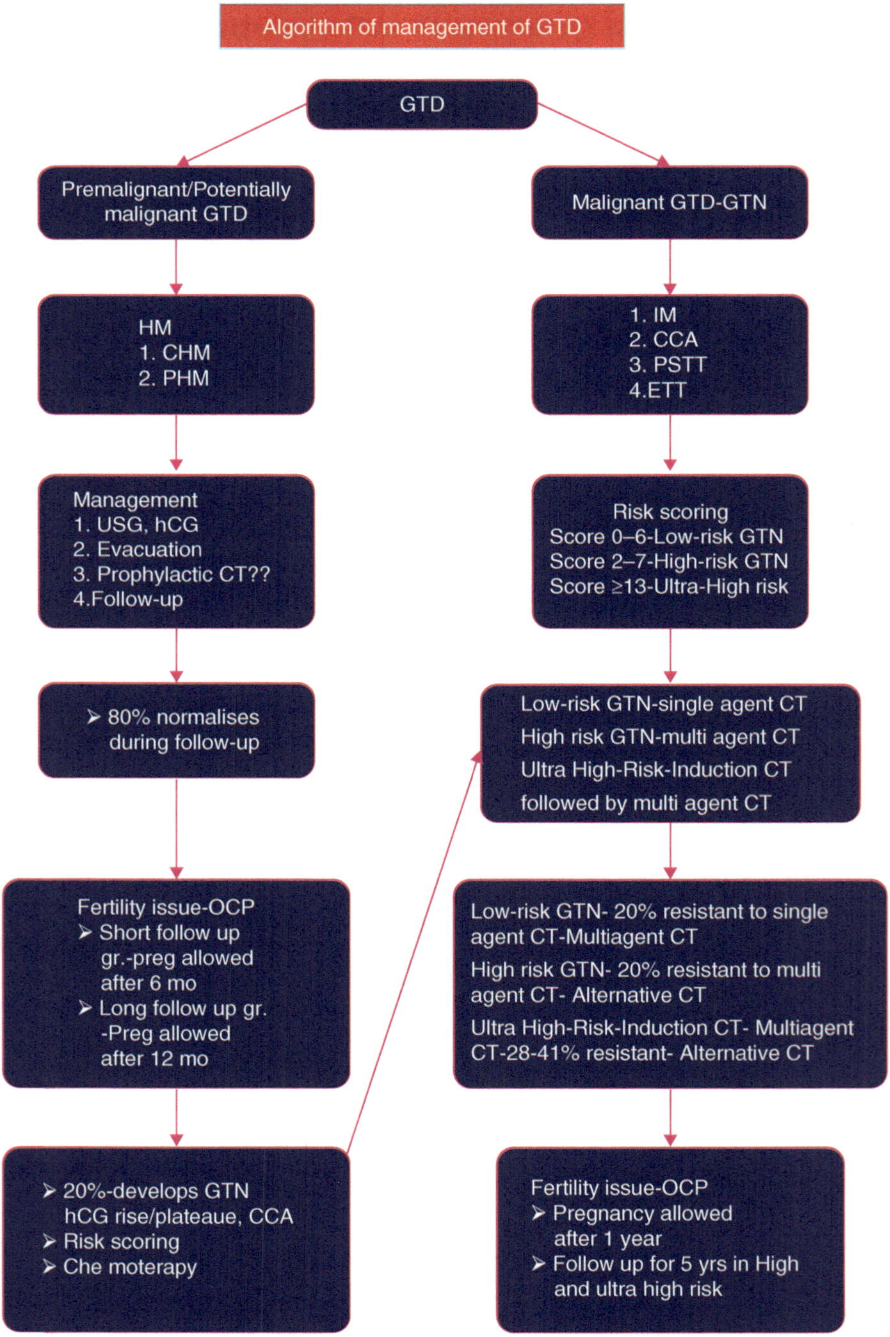

References

1. Lurain JR. Gestational trophoblastic disease: epidemiology, pathology, clinical presentation and diagnosis of gestational trophoblastic disease and management of hydatidiform mole. AM J Obstet Gynecol. 2010;203:531–9.
2. Seckl MJ, Sebire NJ, Berkowitz RS. Gestational trophoblastic disease. Lancet. 2010;376:717–29.
3. Ngan HY, Benders H, Benedet JL, Jones H, Montruccoli GC, Pecorelli S. FIGO 2000 staging and classification. Int J Gynecol Obstet. 2003;83:175–7.
4. Wang Q, Fu J, Hu L, Fang F, Xie L, Chen H, He F, Wu T, Lawrie TA. Prophylactic chemotherapy for hydatidiform mole to prevent gestational trophoblastic neoplasia. Cochrane Database Syst Rev. 2017;9:Art. No.: CD007289.
5. Ngan HY, Seckl MJ, Berkowitz SR, Xiang Y, Sekharan PK, et al. "Update on the diagnosis and management of gestational trophoblastic disease." FIGO CANCER REPORT. Int J Gynecol Obstet. 2018;143(Suppl. 2):79–85.
6. Hammond CB, Borchert LG, Tyrey L, et al. Treatment of metastatic disease; good and poor prognosis. Am J Obstet Gynecol. 1973;115:451–7.
7. Osborne RJ, Filiac VL, Schink JC, Mannel RS, Behbakhi K, et al. Second curettage for low-risk nonmetastatic gestational trophoblastic neoplasia. Obstet Gynecol. 2016 Sept;128(3):535–42.
8. Reda H, Elvira LV, Basem EL-D, Mahammad A, Eman T, et al. Second uterine curettage and number of chemotherapy courses in post molar gestational trophoblastic neoplasia. Obstet Gynecol. 2019;133(5):1024–31.
9. Froeling FEM, Seckl MJ. Uktra high risk gestational trophoblastic neoplasia. TB Gyn Oncol. 2018:1016–20.
10. Santaballa A, Garcıa Y, Herrero A, et al. SEOM clinical guidelines in gestational trophoblastic disease (2017). Clin Transl Oncol. 2018;20:38–46.
11. Tidy J, Seckl M, Hancock BW, on behalf of the Royal College of Obstetricians and Gynaecologists. Management of Gestational Trophoblastic Disease. BJOG 2020.

Epidemiology of Gestational Trophoblastic Diseases

2

Uma Singh, Sabuhi Qureshi, and Manju Lata Verma

Gestational trophoblastic disease (GTD) includes a range of benign and malignant tumors. Amongst these are complete and partial hydatidiform mole, which are benign tumors with malignant potential. The invasive mole, choriocarcinoma, placental site trophoblastic tumor (PSTT), and epithelioid trophoblastic tumor (ETT) are malignant tumors and have varying propensities for local invasion and metastasis. Persistent GTD, also called gestational trophoblastic neoplasia (GTN), includes invasive mole, choriocarcinoma, PSTT, and ETT [1].

All GTNs with the exception of PSTT and ETT, arise from cytotrophoblast and syncytiotrophoblast cells of the villous trophoblast and produce huge amounts of human chorionic gonadotropin (HCG) hormone. PSTT and ETT originate from the intermediate cells of extravillous trophoblast and produce HCG in low amounts [1].

First description of molar pregnancy was given by Hippocrates. Since then, they were associated with high morbidity and mortality owing to serious bleeding and lack of diagnostic modality for early detection. Also, the outcome for GTN was poor before the development of chemotherapy. In the present era, with the advent of safe uterine evacuation methods and effective chemotherapy, GTNs are now some of the most curable of all solid tumors with cure rates of more than 90% even in presence of widespread metastasis [2].

It is difficult to define the incidence and etiologic factors that lead to the development of GTD. Due to lack of uniform case definitions, absence of knowledge about the population at risk, lack of centralized databases, and rarity of the diseases, the data regarding GTN cannot be interpreted [2].

There have been significant changes in women's health issues that have affected the diagnosis and epidemiology of GTD [3].

U. Singh (✉) · M. L. Verma
KG Medical University, Lucknow, India

S. Qureshi
Super Speciality Cancer Institute & Hospital, Lucknow, India

B. Nayak, U. Singh (eds.), *Gestational Trophoblastic Disease*,
https://doi.org/10.1007/978-981-33-4878-3_2

(a) Decrease in birth rate due to availability of reliable contraception has lead to decrease in the incidence of GTD, especially at the extremes of age.
(b) Widespread easy availability of safe methods for termination of pregnancy have led to termination of a large number of conceptions of which some would be GTD. Unless all cases of MTP undergoing termination of pregnancy are subjected to histopathological examination, the diagnosis of GTD will be missed, therefore leading to the reduction in incidence.
(c) With the advent of ultrasonography, GTD is diagnosed much earlier in pregnancy than was seen in pre-ultrasonography era thus reducing the number of undiagnosed GTD presenting at advanced gestation. This has also reduced morbidity and mortality associated with huge hydatidiform moles presenting late in pregnancy.
(d) The early evacuation of abnormal pregnancies now present a diagnostic challenge for the histopathologists to differentiate hydatidiform mole from non-progressive pregnancy (missed or blighted ovum) having hydropic avascular villi.
(e) Availability of hormone assay for HCG has increased the accuracy in diagnosis of GTD and also improvement in follow-up and early detection of GTN.
(f) The advances in medical imaging by CT scan and MRI have led to diagnosing GTN earlier than it was in the era of X-rays. This has impacted upon staging of disease, improvement in management, and follow-up of GTN.
(g) Organized patient follow-up by dedicated centers has led to decrease in the number of patients with seriously advanced GTN as they are picked up early.

2.1 Incidence of H. Mole

The incidence of H. mole shows marked differences across the globe. The incidence is higher in Asia, Africa, and Central America than in the United States, Europe, or Australia. The incidence of HM in Southeast Asia ranges from 1 to 2/1000 pregnancies in Japan and China, to 12/1000 pregnancies in Indonesia and Turkey [3]. In India, the incidence is believed to be 1 in 160 pregnancies [4]. Also, high incidence is reported from Alaska of about 3–4/1000 live births and from Hawaii of about 4–5/1000 live births. Data from North America, Europe, and Oceania reports 0.5–1/1000 pregnancies. Studies from Africa are limited and report between 1 and 3.35/1000 pregnancies. The data from South America is sparse. Some authorities have tried to explain the variation in incidence to risk factors such as maternal age, diet, ethnicity, gravidity, poor social conditions, and pelvic tuberculosis and few have attributed it to differences in prevalence and methodological discrepancies [5–7].

Interestingly, the data of molar pregnancy from South Korea is on a decreasing trend. It was 4.4 cases per 1000 births in the 1960s and which decreased to 1.6 cases per 1000 births in the 1990s, possibly because of improved socioeconomic conditions and dietary changes [5].

2.2 Risk Factors for H. Mole

2.2.1 Maternal Age

There is plenty of evidence available to show that the incidence of HM is increased in teenagers and women over 35 years. Teenagers have a 1.5-fold to twofold increase in risk while women above 35 years have an increased risk and women above 40 years have a five fold or more increase in risk as compared to risk during reproductive years [6]. This is represented as a "J" shaped curve which holds true for different races in different countries. Though the increased risk in the older women is unswervingly high, the effect on the total number of cases of H. Mole is low as the fecundity decreases in this age group. The aging of eggs can also lead to abnormalities in gametogenesis and/or fertilization. This explains higher incidence seen in women >40 years of age but fails to explain the same in teenage population [6].

2.2.2 Diet

Originally deficiency of first-class protein was thought to contribute as an etiological agent for the development of GTD. However, a number of studies have failed to show any relation between the two. This idea was postulated at a time when diet in Southeast Asian countries was poor. In an attempt to evaluate this theory, a laboratory study on 25 patients with H. Mole showed increased levels of serum creatinine and urea concentrations in H. Mole as compared to the levels in controls. At the same time, total protein and serum albumin concentrations were significantly decreased in cases of H. Mole. This was explained by the theory that dietary deficiency leads to catabolism leading in turn, to increased levels of urea and creatinine. These changes, however, may well have been the result of the H. Mole itself. Inappropriate dietary histories were not considered [6]. However, there are few studies on diet which have shown that it can reset the genetic imprint and thus may contribute as a risk factor of GTN. Similarly, deficiency of vitamin A and C has been implicated in genesis of HM.

2.2.3 Gravidity

Increased number of pregnancy has been studied as a risk factor for H. Mole. However, the association appears to be temporal rather than actually being related to gravidity. Studies have failed to show any association between gravidity and H. Mole when the data was corrected for age.

2.2.4 Previous Molar Pregnancies

Women who have had a previous HM appear to be at high risk of having HM again. Relative risk appears to be 5–40 times as compared to the general population. The risk decreases with one or more normal pregnancies following the HM. The risk further increases after a woman has more than one molar pregnancy. After one molar pregnancy, the risk of complete and partial mole rises to 1–2%, after two molar pregnancies the risk of a third molar pregnancy increases to 15–20%. It is also seen that the risk of repeat molar pregnancy is not decreased by change of partner indicating that the trigger mechanism lies in the maternal partner [6].

2.2.5 Genetics

In most cases, complete hydatidiform mole usually arises when an ovum without maternal chromosomes is fertilized by one sperm carrying X chromosome, which then duplicates its DNA, resulting in a 46XX androgenetic karyotype, with all chromosomes derived from the father. Few (10%) of complete moles are 46XY, arising from fertilization by two sperm one having X chromosome and second having Y chromosome. It has also been studied that the nuclear DNA is from the male partner and mitochondrial DNA is from the female partner. Findings from some studies have shown that patients with recurrent disease can have biparental molar pregnancy, i.e., the genetic material being contributed by both partners, rather than typical androgenetic contribution. Genetic studies in such families showed that the related genes responsible are located at chromosome 19q13.3–13.4 with NLRP7 mutations in this region. The mechanism by which these mutations are related to imprinting abnormalities and gestational trophoblastic disease are not known. Clustering of mutations is seen in the leucine-rich region of NLRP7, indicating the importance of normal functioning of this region [8]. Mutation in NLRP7 is also responsible for Familial Recurrent Hydatidiform Mole (FRHM), which is an autosomal recessive condition with biparental CHM (BiCHM).

Partial hydatidiform moles are almost always triploid with both maternal and paternal chromosomes as a result of fertilization of an apparently healthy ovum by two sperms. Diploid partial moles do not exist.

2.2.6 Ethnicity

There is variation in the incidence of HM in different ethnic groups probably because of genetic factors rather than environmental or climatic factors. Genetic factors may lead to higher incidence of abnormal fertilization and/or an increased capacity to permit implantation of a genetically abnormal pregnancy. A Hawaiian study reports the incidence of HM as being highest in Japanese and Philippinos and lowest in whites and native Hawaiians. A study in Alaskan communities has also shown 3–4 times higher incidence rate in comparison to the white population. However, studies from the United States among various racial groups have shown inconsistent results [6].

2.2.7 Contraception

The increased use of contraceptives has decreased the incidence of conceptions at the extremes of reproductive life span and this has affected the incidence of H. Mole. Besides this effect, there was evidence that was suggestive of a link between oral contraceptive intake and increase in the incidence of H. Mole. However, the present evidence does not suggest so and has refuted this theory. Studies observing the association of H. Mole with past use of an intrauterine contraceptive device have shown inconsistent results [6].

2.3 Gestational Trophoblastic Neoplasia

2.3.1 Incidence and Risk Factors

The frequency of choriocarcinoma or placental-site trophoblastic tumor is less well known, since these diseases can arise after any type of pregnancy. Owing to the solid association of H. Mole as a precursor pregnancy with the development of GTN, the country wise incidence of GTN reflects the incidence of H. Mole with statistics for India and Indonesia being the highest at 19.1 and 15.3/100,000 pregnancies respectively and in Southeast Asia, North America, Europe, and Oceania the incidence is between 0.2 and 0.7/100,000 pregnancies. However, a report from Japan has indicated that there has been a reduction in the incidence of choriocarcinoma from 1.6 to 0.3/1,000,000 of population. In this study, the most common antecedent pregnancy is now a term pregnancy [6]. The wide variation in incidence of choriocarcinoma (CC) seen across the globe is because of variation in diagnostic modality used and also because it is a rare tumor. Problems are also encountered due to inconsistencies in case definition and lack of centralized databases. Some use histological parameters for diagnosis and some clinical, radiological, and biochemical parameters. This has led to blurring off of the difference between choriocarcinoma and invasive mole and therefore this group of disease is best referred to as GTN. The two entities are also treated on similar principles [6].

2.3.2 Age

The effect of age on incidence of H. Mole is expected in cases of GTN too owing to the fact that H. Mole is often precursor of choriocarcinoma. Women more than 40 years of age are at high risk of developing post molar GTN as compared to younger women. Although there is no data to support this fact.

2.3.3 Gravidity

The association between gravidity and choriocarcinoma is temporal rather then causal.

2.3.4 History of Previous Molar Pregnancies

There is little doubt that a previous HM predisposes to the development of GTN, consequently a previous HM has been associated with a 1000–2000 times increased risk of choriocarcinoma. The risk is even higher for some morphological and cytogenetic subtypes of the previous HM. In fact, the risk of choriocarcinoma after a complete H. Mole is about 2500 times higher than the risk after a live birth [7].

2.3.5 Genetic

There is no evidence in literature regarding the genetic/chromosomal abnormalities being responsible for choriocarcinoma.

2.3.6 Ethnicity

As mentioned earlier, H. Mole shows higher incidence in certain ethnic groups. A similar pattern is expected for choriocarcinoma too as H. Mole is its precursor. However, the evidence is contradictory. India falls in high incidence group for H.mole and low incidence group for choriocarcinoma. This indicates that some other factor possibly genetic interplays in certain ethnic group and this may be responsible for triggering the malignant change in trophoblast.

2.3.7 Contraception

Some earlier reports suggested an association between oral contraceptive intake after H. Mole and an increased incidence of post molar GTN. This has not been proven in extensive later studies [6].

2.4 Summary

The epidemiology of GTD is not clear. The problems encountered are different methods of data collection, interpretation, and lack of uniform definition and centralized databases. There is a higher incidence of H. Mole in teenagers, women over 35 years, women with history of a previous mole. H. Mole is linked with abnormalities in gametogenesis and/or fertilization. Across the world, Asia witnesses higher incidence and a lower incidence is seen in America and Europe. There is 20% risk of development of GTN after a complete mole. The mechanism for the origin of H. Mole is understood, but very little is known about the triggering process of malignant change in normal and abnormal trophoblast leading to choriocarcinoma and other GTN entities. The surgical and medical advances in gynecology in the last 50 years have reduced the incidence, morbidity, and mortality of GTD.

References

1. Berkowitz R, Goldstein D. Gestational trophoblastic diseases. In: Berek J, Hacker N, editors. Gynaecologic oncology. 6th ed. New York: Wolter Kluvers; 2015. p. 625–48.
2. Lurain RJ. Gestational trophoblastic disease I: epidemiology, pathology, clinical presentation and diagnosis of gestational trophoblastic disease, and management of hydatidiform mole. Am J Obs Gynaecol. 2010;203:6531–9.
3. Bracken MB, Brinton LA, Hayashi K. Epidemiology of hydatidiform mole and choriocarcinoma. Epidemiol Rev. 1984;6:52–75.
4. Daftary SN, Padubidri VG. Trophoblastic diseases. In: Padubidri VG, Daftary SN, editors. Shaw's textbook of gynaecology. 13th ed. New Delhi: Elsevier India Ltd.; 2004. p. 248–59.
5. Seckl MJ, Sebire NJ, Berkowitz RS. Gestational trophoblastic disease. Lancet. 2010;376(9742):717–29.
6. Steigrad SJ. Epidemiology of gestational trophoblastic diseases. Best Pract Res Clin Obstet Gynaecol. 2000;17(6):837–47.
7. Altieri A, Franceschi S, Ferlay J, Smith J, Vecchia CL. Epidemiology and aetiology of gestational trophoblastic diseases. Lancet Oncol. 2003;4:670–6.
8. Stevens FT, Katzorke N, et al. Gestational trophoblastic disorders: an update in 2015. Geburtshilfe Frauenheilkd. 2015;75(10):1043–50.

Genetics and Pathogenesis: A Recent Update

3

Shalini Rajaram and Divya Aggarwal

3.1 Introduction

Gestational trophoblastic diseases (GTDs) include a spectrum of diseases, ranging from premalignant hydatidiform moles (complete and partial) to invasive neoplasms (called gestational trophoblastic neoplasms, GTN) including invasive mole, placental site trophoblastic tumor (PSTT), epithelioid trophoblastic tumor (ETT), and choriocarcinoma. PSTT is derived from implantation site trophoblastic tumor while ETT from chorionic-type intermediate trophoblast [1]. GTDs are unique as these lesions are derived not from patient tissue, but from the conceptus [1].

As a zygote matures into a blastocyst, its peripheral layers differentiate into cytotrophoblast and syncytiotrophoblast. The latter invades into the endometrium and uterine vasculature to form the placental tissue. Uncontrolled proliferation and invasion result in the group of disorders known as GTDs [2].

Partial hydatidiform moles (PHM) are biparental and are formed when a single ovum is fertilized by two (commonly) or rarely, one sperm. Their triploid genome is composed of two sets of paternal chromosomes and a single set of maternal chromosomes with a karyotype of 69, XXX, 69, XXY, or 69, XYY [3]. Occasional cases of tetraploid PHMs are also reported, which appear to result from trispermic fertilization of a single ovum [4].

In contrast, complete hydatidiform moles (CHM) are diploid and uniparental. Kajii and Ohama in 1977 first revealed the androgenetic origin of CHMs [5]. More commonly (in around 80% cases), they occur as a result of duplication of genetic material of a single sperm and in around 20% cases, dispermy is responsible. They have a 46, XX or 46, YY karyotype. Rarely, however, CHMs are biparental. Jacobs

S. Rajaram (✉)
Department of O & G, UCMS, New Delhi, India

D. Aggarwal
Department of Pathology, Postgraduate Institute of Medical Education and Research, Chandigarh, India

B. Nayak, U. Singh (eds.), *Gestational Trophoblastic Disease*,
https://doi.org/10.1007/978-981-33-4878-3_3

et al. in 1982 reported one such case. Biparental CHMs have been found in rare families whose females present with recurrent molar pregnancies [6]. These are known as familial recurrent biparental HMs (FBHMs).

3.2 Maternal DNA in CHMs

Though CHMs are known to be androgenetic, their mitochondrial DNA has been shown to be of maternal origin [7]. Hence theories hypothesizing the fertilization of anucleate eggs by one or two sperms were put forward. However, recent theories suggest post-zygotic diploidization of a triploid conceptus. As per these theories, a biparental zygote is first formed by fertilization of a single egg (M) by one (P1) or two sperms (P1 and P2) resulting in a triploid genome (MP1P1 or MP1P2). This triploid zygote then undergoes abnormal mitosis resulting in 1n, 2n, or 3n derivatives. Since paternal centrioles guide the first mitotic division of a zygote, the presence of two sets of active centrioles often results in abnormal mitoses. So a triploid zygote can result into MP1 (2n) + P2 (1n) or M (1n) + P1P2 (2n) or M + P1 + P2. The 1n outcomes can duplicate their genome to result in androgenetic diploid moles and the 2n P1P2 outcomes can directly produce diploid CHMs. All these would carry maternal mitochondrial DNA as cytoplasmic organelles would have been derived from the egg [3, 8].

The absence of maternal nuclear DNA (more specifically chromosome 11) in CHMs is the basis for p57KIP2 immunostaining. p57KIP2 is transcribed from a paternally imprinted maternally inherited gene CDKN1C [3]. It is expressed in the villous stromal cells of normal placenta. Hence its absence in the villous stromal cells of CHMs can help in differentiating them from PHMs and non-molar pregnancies (which show retained p57KIP2 expresssion) [3]. Occasional cases of PHMs with loss of p57KIP2 due to loss of maternal chromosome 11 have been reported [9]. Retention of maternal chromosome 11 in CHMs can result in positive p57KIP2 immunostaining, which may lead to misdiagnosis [10, 11]. Another paternally imprinted maternally expressed gene is IPL/TSSC3 (imprinted in placenta and liver) whose protein product IPL is absent from cells of CHM [3]. However, since it is not expressed in normal placental cells, its immunostaining, unlike p57KIP2, cannot be used for detection of CHMs.

3.3 Familial CHMs

Familial recurrent biparental hydatidiform moles (FBHM) occur due to mutations in a gene located on 19q13.4, which are inherited in an autosomal recessive manner [12]. These mutations affect the NLRP7 protein, a cytoplasmic protein that belongs to the CATERPILLAR group of proteins [13]. These proteins have an N-terminal pyrin domain, a NACHT domain, and a C-terminal leucine-rich repeat (LRR) domain. Most known mutations in NRLP7 cluster in the LRR domain, indicating that this region may have a crucial role in normal functioning of the protein [3] (Hoffner 2012). The mRNA of NLRP7 has been identified within the cytoplasm of normal oocytes during oogenesis [13]. The precise function of NLRP7 is not clear, however, other proteins of the same family are known to have an important role in inflammation and innate immunity [14]. However, the exact relationship between NLRP7, inflammatory pathways, and HMs is as yet unclear. Abnormal methylation pattern of imprinted genes has been reported in CHMs [15]. Hence, recent research has been aimed at exploring the role of NLRP7 in the process of imprinting.

Imprinting is a reversible epigenetic process that results in silencing the expression of a set of alleles, which can be either maternal or paternal. Transcriptional silencing of one copy of certain genes occurs during gametogenesis. This is achieved by methylation of promotor region [16]. Such genes have only one functional copy in the offspring and any mutation arising within this copy can result in diseases.

Abnormal methylation patterns have been suggested to play a role in familial moles, which could be the result of either inherited abnormalities (involving inherited failure to pass on maternal imprint) or can arise as a result of de novo germline mutations [17, 18]. Owing to the paternal methylation patterns in maternally imprinted genes, FBHMs have a functional overexpression of the paternal genome [15]. The resultant phenotype is similar to androgenetic CHMs (with two copies of paternal chromosomes and no maternal chromosomes). Hayward et al. demonstrated a multilocus maternal imprinting defect in four families with FBHM who had biallelic NLRP7 mutations [19]. These data suggest that at least one of the functions of NLRP7 might be to establish the normal maternal imprinting patterns during embryonic development [13, 20, 21].

In 15 patients with recurrent biparental CHMs, Parry et al. reported the absence of NLRP7 mutations. Three of these women had biallelic mutations of C6orf221, a member of reproduction-related gene cluster on chromosome 6 [22]. They reported no phenotypic differences in CHMs with NLRP7 and C6orf221 mutations [22]. As research on familial CHMs progresses, we are likely to better understand the role of these and possibly other genes in the pathogenesis of BFHMs.

3.4 Genetics of HM

Using microarray analysis, Kato et al. in 2002 demonstrated the expression profile of HMs. They found that genes involved in Ras-MAP kinase, JAK-STAT, and Wnt signalling pathways were upregulated in HMs, suggesting that growth factor or cytokine-mediated signalling pathways may be the mechanisms underlying the trophoblastic proliferation [23]. The downregulated genes include insulin growth factor binding proteins, IL-1, TNF receptor, and CD44 among others [23].

3.5 Role of Maternal and Paternal Sets of Chromosomes

An imbalance in the ratio of maternal and paternal chromosomes occurs in HMs. An excess of paternal chromosomes in the absence of maternal genes results in CHMs that are phenotypically characterized by marked trophoblastic excess and absence of embryo proper. On the other hand, in the presence of maternal chromosomes, an excess of paternal chromosomes produces PHMs which show moderate degree of trophoblastic proliferation and allow for the development of fetus. Interestingly, an excess of maternal chromosomes, as seen in ovarian teratomas, allows for development of embryonic tissues but fails to develop extraembryonic tissue. These findings could suggest that the formation of an embryo proper requires maternal set of chromosomes, while the development of extraembryonic tissues (including trophoblast) is dependent on paternal chromosomes [4]. So when both parents provide equal and appropriate share of their genome, a normal fetus begins to develop.

3.6 Invasive Mole

Both PHMs and CHMs can progress to an invasive mole. These have the potential for local and metastatic spread [24]. Most invasive moles are diploid and are known to be dispermic in origin [25]. A high percentage of tetraploid cells has been reported in invasive moles [26].

3.7 PSTT and ETT

Like most GTNs, genetic data on PSTT and ETT is sparse, however, most PSTTs are reported to be diploid with occasional demonstrating tetraploidy [3]. Few authors have described the karyotype of PSTTs and the abnormalities include absence of Y chromosome, loss of heterozygosity (LOH) 7p11.2, LOH 8p12-p21, and gain of 21q [3]. Xu et al. successfully analyzed three cases of ETT by CGH and found no chromosome gains or losses in any of them [27].

3.8 Choriocarcinoma

Gestational choriocarcinoma is an aggressive tumor that occurs in patients with history of conception, including both molar and non-molar. More than half the cases occur post CHM [28]. The monoallelic genome of a CHM is susceptible to functional inactivation by one-hit kinetics. An additional mechanism of dysregulation of gene expression is by imbalance in the imprinted genes which occurs due to uniparental transmission of genes. These together would result in reduced expression or inactivation of tumor suppressor genes, which predisposes CHMs to malignant transformation [4].

Gestational choriocarcinomas are histologically similar to non-gestational choriocarcinomas, however, they carry a better prognosis and are more chemosensitive than the latter [29]. One plausible explanation is that a part of the genetic material of gestational choriocarcinomas is of paternal origin, hence making them immunogenic and more chemosensitive. They are considered to be partial or complete allografts (containing biparental and uniparental genome, respectively). In contrast, non-gestational choriocarcinomas are host derivatives and hence tend to have poor immunogenicity and response to chemotherapy [3]. Among the gestational choriocarcinomas, those arising from molar pregnancies tend to fare better as compared with those that arise post non-molar conceptions [30].

The genetic makeup of choriocarcinoma has mostly been studied in cell lines and occasionally in fresh tumor tissue. A number of chromosomal alterations including gains, losses, and rearrangements have been detected including deletions of 7p12-q12.2, amplification of 7q21-q31, and loss of 8p12-p21 [31, 32] NECC1 (not expressed on choriocarcinoma 1) gene located on chromosome 4q11-q12 is a tumor suppressor gene, whose expression is reduced in choriocarcinoma cells while it is consistently expressed in normal placental tissue [33].

3.9 Recent Advances

As our understanding of the pathogenetic mechanisms underlying GTDs has improved, the focus has shifted toward application of this knowledge to diagnosis, management, predicting the progression of HMs to GTNs, and understanding chemoresistance. Owing to the rarity of GTNs and paucity of tissue samples (being highly vascular tumors, biopsy is relatively contraindicated in GTNs and most cases directly undergo therapy), most of our understanding is based on research, which has been performed on preserved cell lines [34].

3.10 Genetics in Diagnostics

One of the characteristics used in FIGO risk scoring for GTDs is the interval from index pregnancy in months. Females who develop GTN after a longer interval from the index pregnancy tend to fare worse. However, to conclusively ascertain the index pregnancy becomes difficult in patients with multiple previous pregnancies. A comparison of microsatellite polymorphisms of the tumor with previous pregnancies can help in such cases [34]. Such comparison is also helpful to differentiate gestational from non-gestational choriocarcinomas and a molar versus non-molar origin of a choriocarcinoma, with both the distinctions carrying significant prognostic relevance [3]. Cases that present with a diagnostic uncertainty and where a non-gestational neoplasm is being considered as a differential diagnosis can also be worked up using such genetic analysis tools. This distinction is relevant as GTNs require prompt management with aggressive chemotherapy.

3.11 Predicting Progression to GTN

Approximately 10% CHMs transform to GTNs [35]. The risk of progression is higher for a dispermic CHM in comparison with a monospermic CHM, as suggested by a multitude of studies [25, 36, 37]. However, other studies have contradictory results [38–41]. No significant difference in risk of progression has been reported between BFHMs and androgenetic CHMs [42]. Progression of PHM to GTN is controversial. Case reports of PHMs progressing to GTN do exist in the literature, however, a review of literature shows that the cases which progressed were diploid PHMs and hence could possibly represent misdiagnosed CHMs [41, 43, 44]. It is hence possible that the risk of developing a GTN post PHM is similar to that seen after a non-molar pregnancy [3].

Attempts to determine the factors involved in malignant transformation have been made by comparing the genetic signatures of normal placenta, HMs, and GTNs. However, owing to the rarity of the disease and the paucity of biopsy samples (since a biopsy for confirmation is not done and most cases are treated with chemotherapy without surgery), most research is based on in vitro studies. Activation of oncogenes and inactivation of tumor suppressor genes has been implicated in disease transformation [34]. Upregulation of genes like SET, NANOG, and STAT-3 as well as downregulation of genes including TIMP2, TIMP3, Kiss-1, E-cadherin, DCC-1, APC, beta-catenin, NECC1, caspase 8, caspase 10, and MASPIN have been found to be associated with higher risk of developing GTN from HMs [34].

The role of miRNA has also been explored in progression of HM to GTN. Choriocarcinoma tissues had significant under expression of miR-199b as compared with HMs [34]. Importantly, miRNA expression can be modified by proteins called siRNAs. Forced expression of miRNA-199b has been found to result in a reduction in cellular proliferation in a choriocarcinoma cell line [34].

Another epigenetic event relevant to invasive transformation of HMs is silencing of tumor suppressor genes by methylation of CpG regions. These regions are rich in cytosine and guanine residues and are clustered in the promotor region of various genes. Methylation of CpG islands results in transcriptional silencing of downstream genes. Smith et al. demonstrated that hypermethylation induced silencing of E-cadherin and p16 in HMs can result in invasive transformation [45].

These insights into the pathogenesis of transformation of HMs to GTNs would be clinically relevant when they could be used as biomarkers for identifying those HMs that are at a higher risk of invasive transformation. The current biomarker in use is serum beta hCG (human chorionic gonadotropin). It is a sensitive and relatively noninvasive test that is used for regular follow-up of women with history of HMs. It helps in early identification of cases that are transformed to GTNs. However, at the outset of diagnosis of HM, no current marker exists to identify those women who are likely to develop GTNs. Large prospective clinical trials need to be done on the above genetic markers in the hope of having such a biomarker in the future.

3.12 Genetics of Drug Resistance

GTNs are chemosensitive diseases with nearly 100% survival in FIGO low-risk cases and approximately 87% in high-risk cases [46, 47]. There is a paucity of studies on the exact pathogenetic mechanisms that underlie drug resistance in GTNs. Chen et al. studied cases of 5-fluorouracil and etoposide resistance and found reduced levels of proapoptotic protein PUMA in these cells. On introducing PUMA using an adenovirus vector, an improvement in chemosensitivity was reported [48]. A knowledge of such mutations could theoretically be helpful in identifying at the time of diagnosis, those women whose disease is likely to be chemoresistant.

Recent research on newer drug targets in chemoresistant GTNs has brought into light MAPK (mitogen activated protein kinase) pathway. MAPK is a part of the signalling pathway involved in differentiation and migration. PSTTs demonstrate the active phosphorylated form of MAPK, in contrast to the inactive form found in normal placenta [49]. Treating a PSTT cell line (IST-2) with MAPK inhibitor (CI-1040 and PD 59089) resulted in significant reduction in motility and invasiveness of IST-2 cells. In contrast, the two inhibitors did not have any effect on normal extravillous trophoblastic cells [49].

Other targetable molecules include mTOR (mammalian target of rapamycin), other PI3K family members, and EGFR (epidermal growth factor receptor). These molecules have been found to be upregulated in GTNs including choriocarcinoma and hence they may serve as a therapeutic target [50, 51]. EGFR expression is significantly higher in choriocarcinoma placentae as compared to normal ones with a similar period of gestation [52]. A reduction in EGFR binding sites on choriocarcinoma cells was reported upon exposure to EGFR inhibitors [52]. However, most of this research is based on in vivo cell cultures and clinical trials would serve to provide more definitive results regarding their usefulness as therapy options in chemoresistant GTNs.

3.13 Future Perspective

Many aspects of GTNs remain which need to be explored by future research. To determine and validate biomarkers that can predict the progression of HMs to GTNs, prospective clinical trials need to be carried out. Such studies demand collaborations between the laboratory and clinics. To determine the factors underlying drug resistance and alternative regimens for chemoresistant cases, large clinical trials can be designed. Over longer term, it would be interesting if, at the time of diagnosis, those women can be identified who are at higher risk of progression and resistance to therapy.

References

1. Shih IM, Kurman RJ. Molecular basis of gestational trophoblastic diseases. Curr Mol Med. 2002;2(1):1–12.
2. Candelier JJ. The hydatidiform mole. Cell Adh Migr. 2016;10(1–2):226–35.
3. Hoffner L, Surti U. The genetics of gestational trophoblastic disease: a rare complication of pregnancy. Cancer Genet. 2012;205(3):63–77.
4. Matsuda T, Wake N. Genetics and molecular markers in gestational trophoblastic disease with special reference to their clinical application. Best Pract Res Clin Obstet Gynaecol. 2003;17(6):827–36.
5. Kajii T, Ohama K. Androgenetic origin of hydatidiform mole. Nature. 1977;268:633–4.

6. Jacobs PA, Hunt PA, Matsuura JS, et al. Complete and partial hydatidiform mole in Hawaii: cytogenetics, morphology and epidemiology. Br J Obstet Gynaecol. 1982;89:258–66.
7. Wallace DC, Surti U, Adams CW, et al. Complete moles have paternal chromosomes but maternal mitochondrial DNA. Hum Genet. 1982;61:145–7.
8. Golubovsky MD. Postzygotic diploidization of triploids as a source of unusual cases of mosaicism, chimerism and twinning. Hum Reprod. 2003;18:236–42.
9. Hoffner L, Parks WT, Swerdlow SH, et al. Simultaneous detection of imprinted gene expression (p57(KIP2)) and molecular cytogenetics (FICTION) in the evaluation of molar pregnancies. J Reprod Med. 2010;55:219–28.
10. Fisher RA, Nucci MR, Thaker HM, et al. Complete hydatidiform mole retaining a chromosome 11 of maternal origin: molecular genetic analysis of a case. Mod Pathol. 2004;17:1155–60.
11. McConnell TG, Norris-Kirby A, Hagenkord JM, et al. Complete hydatidiform mole with retained maternal chromosomes 6 and 11. Am J Surg Pathol. 2009;33:1409–15.
12. Moglabey YB, Kircheisen R, Seoud M, El Mogharbel N, Van den Veyver I, Slim R. Genetic mapping of a maternal locus responsible for familial hydatidiform moles. Hum Mol Genet. 1999;8:667–71.
13. Wang CM, Dixon PH, Decordova S, et al. Identification of 13 novel *NLRP7* mutations in 20 families with recurrent hydatidiform mole; missense mutations cluster in the leucine-rich region. J Med Genet. 2009;46(8):569–75.
14. Ogura Y, Sutterwala FS, Flavell RA. The inflammasome: first line of the immune response to cell stress. Cell. 2006;126(4):659–62.
15. Judson H, Hayward BE, Sheridan E, et al. A global disorder of imprinting in the human female germ line. Nature. 2002;416:539–42.
16. Kumar V, Abbas AK, Aster JC. Robbins basic pathology. 10th ed. Philadelphia, PA: Elsevier; 2018.
17. Judson H, Hayward BE, Sheridan E, Bonthron DT. A global disorder of imprinting in the human female germ line. Nature. 2002;416:539–42.
18. El-Maarri O, Seoud M, Rivière JB, et al. Patients with familial biparental hydatidiform moles have normal methylation at imprinted genes. Eur J Hum Genet. 2005;13:486–90.
19. Hayward BE, De Vos M, Talati N, et al. Genetic and epigenetic analysis of recurrent hydatidiform mole. Hum Mutat. 2009;30(5):E629–39.
20. Kou YC, Shao L, Peng HH, et al. A recurrent intragenic genomic duplication, other novel mutations in *NLRP7* and imprinting defects in recurrent biparental hydatidiform moles. Mol Hum Reprod. 2008;14(1):33–40.
21. El-Maarri O, Slim R. Familial hydatidiform molar pregnancy: the germline imprinting defect hypothesis? Curr Top Microbiol Immunol. 2006;301:229–41.
22. Parry DA, Logan CV, Hayward BE, et al. Mutations causing familial biparental hydatidiform mole implicate C6orf221 as a possible regulator of genomic imprinting in the human oocyte. Am J Hum Genet. 2011;89:451–8.
23. Kato H, Terao Y, Ogawa M, et al. Growth-associated gene expression profiles by microarray analysis of trophoblast of molar pregnancies and normal villi. Int J Gynecol Pathol. 2002;21:255–60.
24. Lurain JR. Gestational trophoblastic disease II: classification and management of gestational trophoblastic neoplasia. Am J Obstet Gynecol. 2011;204:11–8.
25. Wake N, Seki T, Fujita H, et al. Malignant potential of homozygous and heterozygous complete moles. Cancer Res. 1984;44:1226–30.
26. Yang YH, Kwak HM, Park TK, et al. Comparative cytogenetic and clinicopathologic studies on gestational trophoblastic neoplasia, especially hydatidiform mole. Yonsei Med J. 1986;27:250–60.
27. Xu ML, Yang B, Carcangiu ML, et al. Epithelioid trophoblastic tumor: comparative genomic hybridization and diagnostic DNA genotyping. Mod Pathol. 2009;22:232–8.

28. Palmer JR. Advances in the epidemiology of gestational trophoblastic disease. J Reprod Med. 1994;39:155–62.
29. Cheung AN, Zhang HJ, Xue WC, et al. Pathogenesis of choriocarcinoma: clinical, genetic and stem cell perspectives. Future Oncol. 2009;5:217–31.
30. Kohorn EI. Negotiating a staging and risk factor scoring system for gestational trophoblastic neoplasia. A progress report. J Reprod Med. 2002;47:445–50.
31. Ahmed MN, Kim K, Haddad B, et al. Comparative genomic hybridization studies in hydatidiform moles and choriocarcinoma: amplification of 7q21-q31 and loss of 8p12-p21 in choriocarcinoma. Cancer Genet Cytogenet. 2000;116:10–5.
32. Matsuda T, Sasaki M, Kato H, et al. Human chromosome 7 carries a putative tumor suppressor gene(s) involved in choriocarcinoma. Oncogene. 1997;15:2773–81.
33. Asanoma K, Kato H, Inoue T, et al. Analysis of a candidate gene associated with growth suppression of choriocarcinoma and differentiation of trophoblasts. J Reprod Med. 2004;49:617–26.
34. Alifrangis C, Seckl MJ. Genetics of gestational trophoblastic neoplasia: an update for the clinician. Future Oncol. 2010;6(12):1915–23.
35. Sebire NJ, Seckl MJ. Gestational trophoblastic disease: current management of hydatidiform mole. BMJ. 2008;337:1193.
36. Kajii T, Kurashige H, Ohama K, et al. XY and XX complete moles: clinical and morphologic correlations. Am J Obstet Gynecol. 1984;150:57–64.
37. Wake N, Fujino T, Hoshi S, et al. The propensity to malignancy of dispermic heterozygous moles. Placenta. 1987;8:319–26.
38. Fisher RA, Lawler SD. Heterozygous complete hydatidiform moles: do they have a worse prognosis than homozygous complete moles? Lancet. 1984;2:51.
39. Mutter GL, Pomponio RJ, Berkowitz RS, et al. Sex chromosome composition of complete hydatidiform moles: relationship to metastasis. Am J Obstet Gynecol. 1993;168:1547–51.
40. Cheung AN, Sit AS, Chung LP, et al. Detection of heterozygous XY complete hydatidiform mole by chromosome in situ hybridization. Gynecol Oncol. 1994;55:386–92.
41. van de Kaa CA, Schijf CP, de Wilde PC, et al. Persistent gestational trophoblastic disease: DNA image cytometry and interphase cytogenetics have limited predictive value. Mod Pathol. 1996;9:1007–14.
42. Fisher RA, Hodges MD. Genomic imprinting in gestational trophoblastic disease review. Placenta. 2003;24:S111–8.
43. Kaneki E, Kobayashi H, Hirakawa T, et al. Incidence of postmolar gestational trophoblastic disease in androgenetic moles and the morphological features associated with low risk postmolar gestational trophoblastic disease. Cancer Sci. 2010;101:1717–21.
44. Niemann I, Hansen ES, Sunde L. The risk of persistent trophoblastic disease after hydatidiform mole classified by morphology and ploidy. Gynecol Oncol. 2007;104:411–5.
45. Smith HO. Gestational trophoblastic disease epidemiology and trends. Clin Obstet Gynecol. 2003;46(3):541–56.
46. McNeish IA, Strickland S, Holden L, et al. Low-risk persistent gestational trophoblastic disease: outcome after initial treatment with low-dose methotrexate and folinic acid from 1992 to 2000. J Clin Oncol. 2002;20(7):1838–44.
47. Bower M, Newlands ES, Holden L, et al. EMA/CO for high-risk gestational trophoblastic tumors: results from a cohort of 272 patients. J Clin Oncol. 1997;15(7):2636–43.
48. Chen Y, Qian H, Wang H, et al. Ad-PUMA sensitizes drug-resistant choriocarcinoma cells to chemotherapeutic agents. *Gynecol*. Oncology. 2007;107(3):505–12.
49. Kobel M, Pohl G, Schmitt WD, Hauptmann S, Wang TL, IEM S. Activation of mitogen-activated protein kinase is required for migration and invasion of placental site trophoblastic tumor. Am J Pathol. 2005;167(3):879–85.
50. Mparmpakas D, Zacharides E, Foster H, Harvey A. Expression of *mTOR* and downstream signalling components in the JEG-3 and BeWo human placental choriocarcinoma cell lines. Int J Mol Med. 2010;25(1):65–9.

51. Tuncer ZS, Vegh GL, Fulop V, Genest DR, Mok SC, Berkowitz RS. Expression of epidermal growth factor receptor-related family products in gestational trophoblastic diseases and normal placenta and its relationship with development of postmolar tumor. Gynecol Oncol. 2000;77(3):389–93.
52. Sarkar S, Kacinski BM, Kohorn EI, et al. Demonstration of myc and ras oncogene expression by hybridization in situ in hydatidiform mole and in the BeWo choriocarcinoma cell line. Am J Obstet Gynecol. 1986;154:390–3.

Human Chorionic Gonadotropin

4

Ashok Kumar Padhy, Deepika Dash, and Richi Khandelwal

4.1 Introduction

HCG is a hormone unique to gestation, however, it may be raised in other pathological states as well. Human chorionic gonadotropin (hCG) is a placental hormone secreted after implantation and is commonly detected by urine gravindex test. It interacts with the LHCG receptor of the ovary and maintains the corpus luteum during initial weeks of pregnancy. It is also produced by most of the trophoblastic tumors where the serial quantitative detection with rise and fall gives information about the course of the disease, prognosis, treatment, treatment response, and recurrence. Various levels of rise are observed in gestational trophoblastic disease and very very high level in its malignant counterpart Gestational Trophoblastic Neoplasia, including Choriocarcinoma. It is secreted mainly by the syncytiotrophoblasts soon after implantation, though also secreted in small amounts by the anterior pituitary. hCG is solely responsible for maintaining pregnancy before progesterone takes over at 12 weeks of gestation. There are various different forms of hCG that have been identified, although the function of each type is yet to be defined. It is imperative that whatever information is available be utilized for the accurate characterization of hCG-associated lesions [1].

This chapter would focus on the different types of hCG and their biological significance.

The original version of this chapter was revised (third author name in this chapter was corrected as Richi Khandelwal). The correction to this chapter can be found at https://doi.org/10.1007/978-981-33-4878-3_19

A. K. Padhy (✉)
AHPGIC, Cuttack, India

D. Dash · R. Khandelwal
Department of Gynaec Oncology, AHPGIC, Cuttack, India

B. Nayak, U. Singh (eds.), *Gestational Trophoblastic Disease*,
https://doi.org/10.1007/978-981-33-4878-3_4

4.2 Structure

HCG is composed of two subunits alpha (α) and beta (β) held together by non-covalent hydrophobic and ionic bonds and contain a total of eight carbohydrate side chains [1]. It is composed of 237 amino acids (92 in α and 145 in β) and the molecular weight is approximately 36 KDa. The alpha-subunit is homologous to that of TSH, LH, and FSH whereas the β-subunit has 80–85% homology to LH. The difference between β-subunit of LH and hCG is in 24 amino acids in the carboxyl-terminal peptide (CTP), which is unique to hCG. Consequent to this sharing, there is cross-reactivity between the two molecules; also the longer half-life of hCG compared to LH is attributed to the four glycosylated serine residues in the CTP. Thirty percent of the weight of hCG is due to the eight carbohydrate side chains. It is the changes in these side chains, which result in three different types of hCG isoforms: regular hCG, sulfated hCG, and hyperglycosylated hCG [2, 3]. The alpha-subunit is encoded by a single gene at chromosome 6q12–q21 while the β-subunit is encoded by six non-allelic genes located at chromosome 19q13.32 [4].

4.3 Production

Naturally, it is produced in the human placenta by the syncytiotrophoblast. hCG peaks at 10 weeks of gestation then plateaus as gestation advances. So, it is likely to be raised wherever syncytiotrophoblast is present, for example—gestational trophoblastic neoplasia and germ cell tumors with trophoblastic elements. In consensus with the site of production, 15–20% of seminiferous testicular tumors and 40–50% non-seminiferous testicular tumors secrete hCG. Traditionally for pharmacological use, it has been extracted from the urine of pregnant woman, but a more purified form can be produced using genetically modified techniques, which is free from any contamination and is thus, much safer to use.

4.4 Metabolism

It is primarily metabolized by the liver and 20% is excreted by the kidneys. The half-life of injectable HCG and that produced during pregnancy differs slightly as the purified injected forms get partly denatured during processing. Also, there are differences in clearance rates of the alpha and β-subunit with the latter having a longer half-life owing to differences in glycosylation. The major byproduct of hCG metabolism is the β-core fragment (cf). More than 99% of HCGβcf is formed in the kidneys during renal excretion. After injection of urinary HCG, HCGβ, or recombinant HCG (rHCG), peak concentrations of HCGβcf occur approximately 6 h after the HCG peak in urine [5, 6].

4.5 Functions

- Immunomodulation—hCG protects the developing fetus from the immune system of the mother [7, 8] hCG has a high negative charge, so repels the immune cells of the mother, protecting the fetus during the first trimester. hCG is a link in the development of peritrophoblastic immune tolerance, which facilitates the trophoblast invasion responsible for development of suitable environment in endometrium.
- Implantation—helps in trophoblastic invasion.
- Early pregnancy—hCG binds to its receptor of the ovary and maintains the corpus luteum up to 12 weeks till the placenta takes over. It has also been suggested that hCG levels are linked to the severity of morning sickness or Hyperemesis gravidarum in pregnant women.
- Ovulation induction—Because of its similarity to LH, hCG is used clinically to trigger ovulation in ART procedures.
- Male pseudo-hermaphroditism—to increase testosterone production.

4.6 Forms of hCG

Various isoforms of hCG are known like total hCG, intact hCG, free β-subunit hCG, hyperglycosylated hCG, nicked hCG, alpha hCG, and pituitary hCG [2, 3].

Only the intact, hyperglycosylated, and pituitary variants have been described in detail in the following text.

4.6.1 Intact hCG

This is the main form of hCG associated with the majority of pregnancy and in noninvasive molar pregnancies. This is produced in the trophoblast cells of the placental tissue.

4.6.2 Free β-subunit hCG

The difference between free β-subunit and β-subunit is that the free β-subunit is a hyperglycosylated variant of the β-subunit of hCG. Increased levels are seen in hydatidiform mole, choriocarcinoma, and non-trophoblastic cancers of all primaries. It has an important role to play in non-gestational neoplasm by serving as a promoter of malignant transformation thereby leading to poor clinical outcome [6]. Hence, targeted antibody directed to this specific subunit can help in controlling the disease. Owing to this knowledge, efforts are ongoing to develop a vaccine containing β-subunit for treating non-gestational malignancies.

4.6.3 Hyperglycosylated hCG

Glycosylation of hCG occurs by any sequential addition of carbohydrate side chains just before release of the assembled dimmer, it is not only of structural importance but has an important functional role as well. Glycosylated hCG has a different rate of clearance from the body apart from a unique biological action. This process of glycosylation of hCG is variable and this leads to the production of a variety of glycoforms and only some have been understood till now. The glycosylation of tumor-derived hCG is also highly variable with increased amount of abnormal glycans and hence referred to as hyperglycosylated. This hyperglycosylated hCG is recognized by a specific antibody, B152. This form of hCG could serve as a biomarker of an invasive trophoblastic phenotype [9].

4.6.4 Pituitary hCG

Pituitary hCG or sulfated hCG is another form secreted by the pituitary gland. It contains half of sialic acid as that of intact hCG and some of the glycans are sulfated and hence the name. It is relatively less active than hCG. Its concentration increases during menopause and is about 0.5–5 IU/L for most women. Levels have also been found to be raised post chemotherapy. Although it is increased at low levels only, but it is important to differentiate from early pregnancy or malignant disease.

4.7 Clinical Importance of Different Isoforms

4.7.1 Pregnancy

Intact HCG comprises more than 95% of total hCG in maternal circulation during the few weeks of pregnancy. The free alpha-subunit also comprises less than 10% in the first trimester but increases throughout pregnancy to become 30–60% at term. The free β-subunit is less than 10% in very early pregnancy and is 0.5–2% after the eighth week. Urinary concentrations of free β-subunit are, however, higher (9–40%) [10]. Hyperglycosylated hCG is the predominant form of hCG in early pregnancy in serum and urine. Low levels are seen in preeclampsia and associated with pregnancy loss [11, 12]. It has also been considered as a marker of normally functioning invasive extra villous cytotrophoblast necessary for implantation. Hence, ineffective invasion is usually seen due to insufficient hyperglycosylated hCG. High levels seen in Down syndrome are used as a screening method in high-risk pregnancy [13].

The most important form in urine is composed of hCG β-subunit core fragment hCG. It is the final product of hCG metabolism. However, it is not recognized by the many available commercially available hCG assays. Nicked forms are more rapidly cleared than intact heterodimer and moreover, due to their relatively higher concentrations, they are more abundant in urine than serum. The proportion of the nicked silenced) and p57 is expressed from the maternal allele. p57 serves as a marker of genetic imprinting and is not implicated in the pathogenesis of molar gestation. This immunostain using paternity as the basis has primary utility in separating CHM from other types of specimens. However, further separation between positively staining specimens including PHM and non-molar specimens is limited (Fig. 5.2).

Staining is interpreted in the nucleus of villous cytotrophoblasts, villous stromal cells, intermediate trophoblasts, and maternal decidua. Nuclear staining of intermediate trophoblasts and maternal decidua serves as the internal control for p57 and its staining is required in all types of specimens before interpretation in the villous cells.

Apparent expression in villous intermediate trophoblastic cells is seen even in the diandric CHM due to mechanism of "epigenetic relaxation," which is an expression from paternal allele owing to heterogenous paternal imprinting patterns across the genome, in the absence of maternal allele.

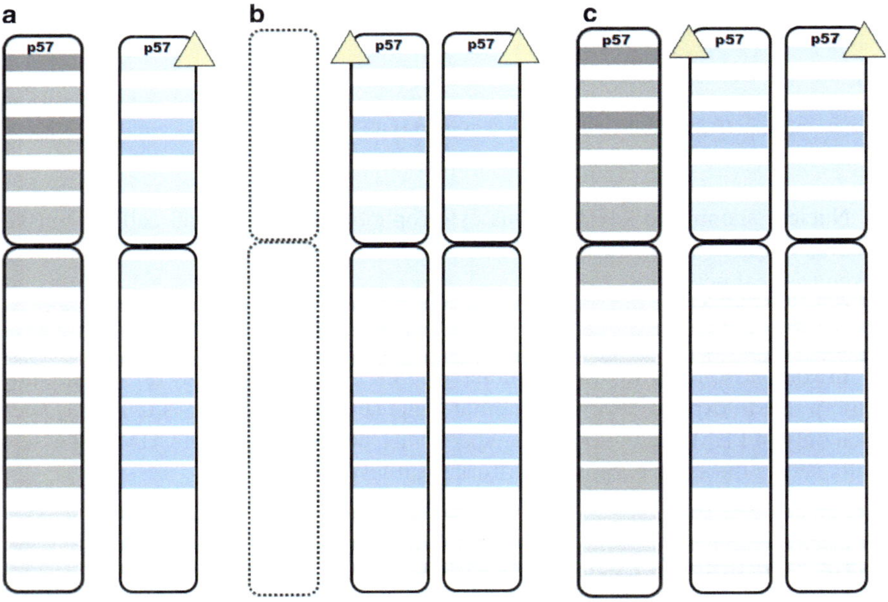

Fig. 5.2 Schematic representation of the genetic principle of p57 expression in non-molar and molar gestation. (**a**) Normal/non-molar gestation with biparental profile and imprinted p57 paternal allele results in p57 expression from the maternal allele; (**b**) Complete hydatidiform mole with two imprinted p57 paternal alleles results in absence of p57 expression due to the absence of maternal allele; (**c**) Partial hydatidiform mole results in expression of p57 from the maternal complement despite the presence of two paternally derived methylated copies of p57. ▲ (filled triangle): Trimethyl groups, addition of which leads to genetic imprinting of p57 gene

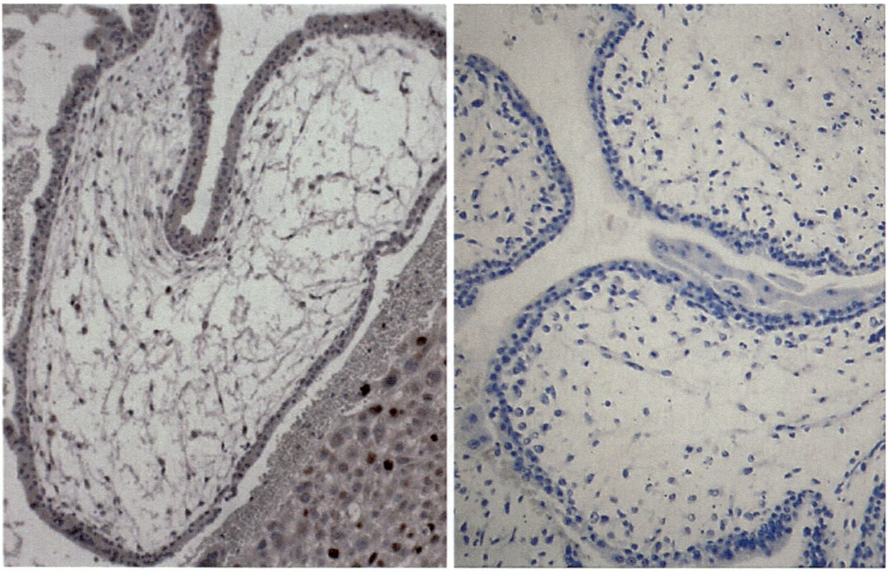

Fig. 5.3 p57 expression in CHM. Negative staining in cytotrophoblasts and villous stromal cells. Intermediate trophoblasts and decidual stromal cells serve as internal control and show positive nuclear staining (Reproduced with permission from Hui P, 2011, Springer)

Nuclear staining in <10% villous cytotrophoblasts and stromal cells is considered as negative while diffuse (>50%) nuclear staining is positive and 10–50% is taken as focal positivity.

Complete hydatiform moles show absence (or very limited) staining for p57 due to lack of maternal allele of the gene (Fig. 5.3).

In comparison, PHM and non-molar specimens, however, show diffuse staining pattern due to expression from maternal allele (Fig. 5.4). Focal positivity has been seen only in PHM and in non-molar specimens, however, never in CHM and essentially serves the same purpose as diffuse positivity [14].

5.3.2 Variants of Positive Staining

5.3.2.1 Discordant Pattern of Staining

The staining pattern is considered discordant when the villous trophoblastic cells and villous stromal cells show different staining i.e, either positively stained trophoblastic cells and negative stromal cells or vice versa. This pattern of staining is characteristic of *androgenetic/biparental mosaic conceptions* with p57-representing the androgenetic component and the p57+, the biparental component [15–17].

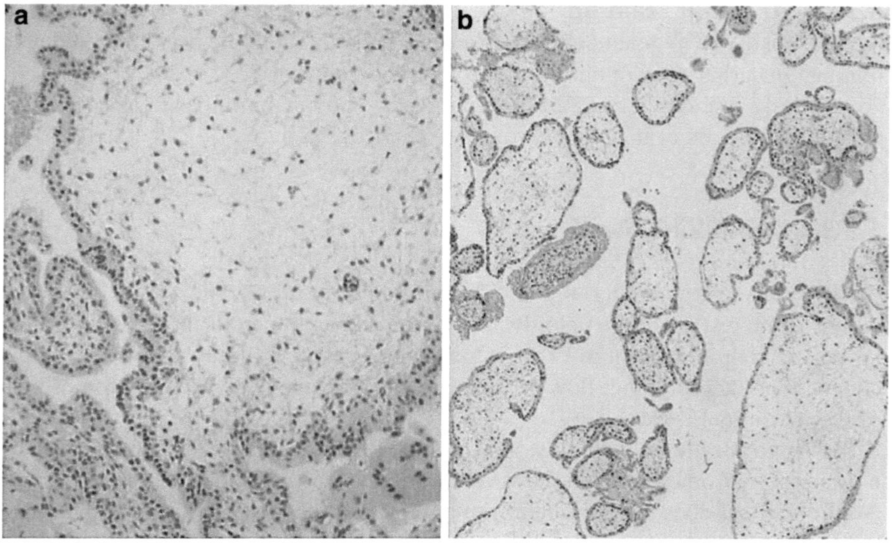

Fig. 5.4 p57 expression in PHM (**a**) and diploid non-molar gestation with abnormal villus morphology (**b**) Both types of specimens although genetically distinct show similar staining pattern with diffuse positive staining in cytotrophoblasts, intermediate trophoblasts, villous stromal cells, and decidual stromal cells (Reproduced with permission from Hui P, 2011, Springer)

5.3.2.2 Divergent Pattern of Staining

This pattern of staining encountered in *twin gestation with complete mole and a non-molar gestation* results from an admixture of two populations of morphologically dissimilar villi with one set showing complete absence of staining and the other set showing diffuse positivity. The p57- villi are derived from androgenetic CHM and p57+ villi represent biparental non-molar abortus.

In either the absence of p57 testing or failure to recognize the divergent patterns of p57 staining, these cases will be erroneously classified as partial mole based on morphology alone [18].

5.3.2.3 Divergent-Discordant Pattern of Staining

This pattern of staining is seen in *androgenetic/biparental mosaic conception with a molar component*, with discordant p57 staining (usually positive staining in villous cytotrophoblasts and negative staining in villous stromal cells) in the non-molar androgenetic/biparental component and completely negatively stained villi representing the complete mole [14].

Morphologically they consist of two populations of villi, mosaic villi without trophoblastic proliferation and androgenetic villi with trophoblastic proliferation. Without the correct interpretation of the divergent-discordant pattern of p57 immunostaining, they may be misclassified as partial mole. Furthermore, STR genotyping in these cases yields complex data, especially if the tissue is not adequately microdissected for PCR.

5.3.2.4 Aberrant Staining

Diffuse positivity in genetically confirmed CHM may rarely be encountered due to retained maternal copy of chromosome 11, encoding for p57 [19, 20].

Similarly rare cases of PHM showing loss of p57 staining have been reported, attributable to loss of maternal chromosome 11 [21, 22].

5.3.3 DNA Ploidy Analysis

Ploidy refers to the number of haploid sets (23 chromosomes) present in cell population of interest, with aneuploidy referring to deviation from the normal diploid karyotype. Triploidy seen in PHM is the genetic basis for ploidy analysis by either conventional karyotyping, flow cytometry, digital image analysis, or chromosomal enumeration by FISH.

By demonstration of triploidy, it is possible to separate out PHM from CHM and non-molar hydropic gestation, however, it does not further delineate between them. Additionally, it does not provide information regarding the paternal contribution to the triploid karyotype and thus cannot distinguish between PHM and triploid digynic monoandric non-molar gestation.

Conventional karyotyping is the most accurate among the different methods available for the determination of ploidy, however, requires fresh chorionic villous tissue and in vitro cell cultures. Flow cytometry is the most frequently used method using tissue specimens including paraffin-embedded formalin-fixed tissue. When FFPE samples are used, effects of fixative used and fixation time along with contaminating DNA have significant impact on peak lengths and coefficient of variation which may lead to misinterpretation of ploidy.

Digital image analysis (DIA) uses Fuelgen DNA stain in contrast to fluorescent binding dyes in FCM and the amount of light transmitted through the test slide is compared with the light transmitted through the control slide to estimate the ploidy of the test cell population.

5.3.3.1 Fluorescent In Situ Hybridization (FISH)

Chromosomal enumeration using probes for multiple loci are comparably informative as conventional karyotype and have largely replaced the same, as they can be conveniently performed on FFPE tissue.

Tests exploring the parental source of chromosomes such as polymorphic deletion probe FISH (PDP-FISH) based on pericentromeric chromosome heteromorphism require fresh tissue samples like conventional karyotyping and require adequate validation studies before considering them for diagnostic utility [23].

5.3.4 DNA Genotyping by PCR Amplification of STR Loci

Genotyping identifies the genetic variation between any two individuals within the same species. Short tandem repeats are highly polymorphic microsatellite loci comprising of variable number (2–10) of nucleotide repeats, prevalent in the non-coding regions. Determination of the number of repeats at specific STR loci establishes the unique genetic profile for an individual. Despite the possibility of shared alleles at some loci, the allelic pattern across several loci remains unique for every individual. STR polymorphism genotyping has been a useful genetic marker in forensics, paternity testing, and its utility can be extrapolated for diagnosis in GTDs.

For analysis in GTDs, the allelic patterns at each STR locus for maternal decidual tissue and villous tissue are compared in pairs. The parental source and ploidy thus analyzed (in pairs) distinguish between CHM, PHM, and non-molar specimens.

Microdissection of the sample from FFPE tissue, isolating pure maternal decidual tissue and villous tissue into two PCR tubes with minimal cross contamination is of vital importance and serves as a prerequisite condition for accurate analysis.

Commercially available STR genotyping PCR kits include at least 13 loci required for the CODIS (Combined DNA index system) loci, with AmpFlSTR® Identifiler™ including two additional loci and Amelogenin, a gender determining locus in a single multiplex PCR reaction using fluorescently labelled, loci specific primers.

Identification of informative STR loci or unique paternal alleles by comparing allelic positions at each STR locus is the key step for interpretation of STR genotyping. Although alleles may be shared between parental sources, due to limited number of alleles at specific loci, it is unlikely that the alleles are shared at all STR loci (Fig. 5.5).

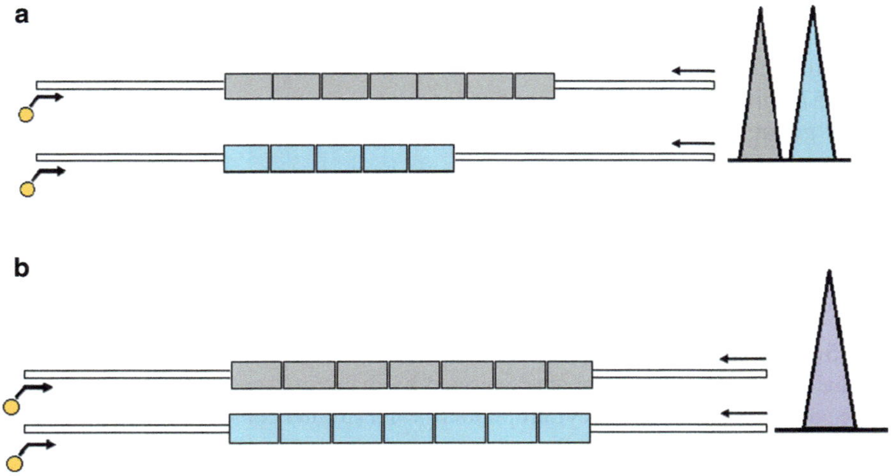

Fig. 5.5 Principle of STR loci amplification by PCR. Fluorescent probes labelling specific STR loci result in two separate peaks on capillary electrophoresis following amplification of heterogenous maternal and paternal alleles (**a**), or a single peak in case the allele is shared among both the parental complements (**b**)

In the absence of a unique paternal allele at a locus, the copy number indicated by the PCR allelic height may be used in comparison with the adjacent allele for ploidy analysis.

Alleles from the maternal decidua are compared with alleles from the villi which are considered to be paternal/nonmaternal or possibly paternal in case of shared alleles. The relative copy number/dosage of an allele at each STR locus in the pair can be determined by calculating a mathematical ratio using either the peak height or the peak area of the two alleles. Alleles present in equal dosage result in a ratio of 1:1 whereas an allele present in double dosage relative to the other, results in a ratio of 2:1.

Uniform concordance of genetic alterations is often observed at all loci for the diagnosis of molar gestation. Discordant findings at isolated loci are particularly observed in case of loss or gain of that allele due to chromosomal aberrations and require careful interpretation of other loci before erroneous interpretation.

5.3.5 Genotypic STR Polymorphism PCR in Molar Gestation and Non-Molar Hydropic Gestation

5.3.5.1 Complete Hydatidiform Mole

Complete hydatidiform moles comprise androgenetic p57-ve villous cytotrophoblasts and stromal cells with diploid diandric karyotype. They show a single nonmaternal allele in double dosage at informative STR loci on genotyping, as they are commonly monospermic (Fig. 5.6).

5.3.5.2 False Negative Probability

Rare cases of biparental CHM, which have morphology and complete absent staining of p57 as in classic diandric CHM show a biparental diploid karyotype. Therefore, the genotyping results have been interpreted in the light of morphology and p57 staining to avoid misclassification of this entity as diploid biparental non-molar gestation.

5.3.5.3 False Positive Probability

If genotyping alone is interpreted, without morphologic and p57 immunostain correlation and in the absence of adequate clinical history in donor egg conception, non-molar gestations may be misclassified as androgenetic CHM.

5.3.5.4 Partial Hydatiform Mole

Partial hydatiform moles are characterized by diandric monogynic triploid karyotype and show p57+ villous cytotrophoblasts and stromal cells. On genotyping, they either show three unique allelic patterns at informative loci (two paternal and one maternal) in equal dosage when heterozygous/dispermic or two unique allelic patterns with the paternal allele in double dosage and an allelic ratio of 2:1 in monospermic/homozygous partial moles (Fig. 5.7).

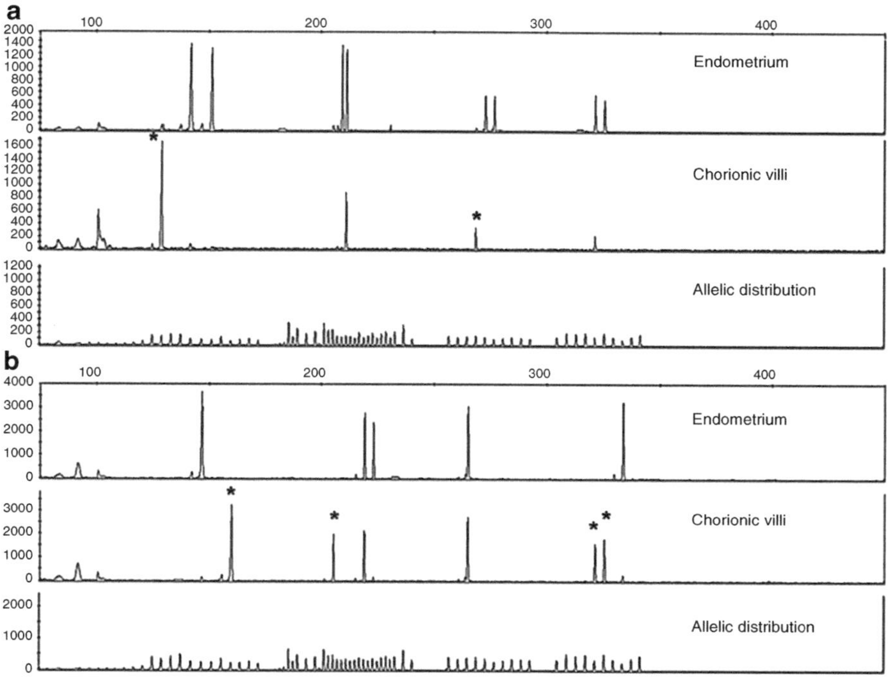

Fig. 5.6 STR genotyping of CHM (4 of 15 STR loci of AmpFlSTR Identifiler are shown: CSF1PO, D7S820, D8S1179, and D21S11). A homozygous complete mole (**a**) harbors exclusively paternal alleles in the villous tissue at all loci. A heterozygous complete mole (**b**) shows exclusively paternal alleles in the villous tissue at all loci with identifiable two distinct paternal alleles at some loci. The unique paternal alleles are indicated by an asterisk (Reproduced with permission from Hui P, 2011, Springer)

5.3.5.5 Non-Molar Gestation with Digynic Monoandric Karyotype

An allelic ratio of 2:1 without the presence of two unique paternal alleles at informative loci points toward this diagnosis.

5.3.5.6 Non-Molar Gestation with Chromosomal Alterations in Number

Abnormal villous morphology related to trisomies shows allelic ratios of 2:1 on genotyping, if the STR loci on the chromosome involved are included in the PCR kit and the allelic pattern and the number of loci involved depend on the parental source and the number of chromosomes involved. However, they show balanced biparental alleles at other loci.

In the absence of sufficient informative STR loci, if the extra chromosomes are paternal in origin, trisomies (individual, double, or rarely multiple) may be erroneously interpreted as diandric triploid PHM.

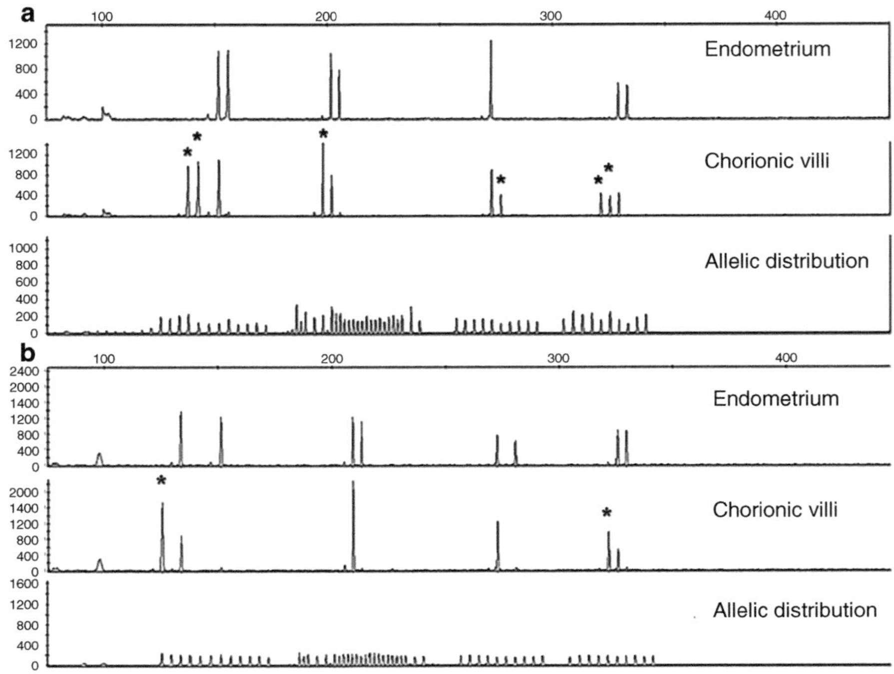

Fig. 5.7 STR genotyping of partial hydatidiform mole (4 of 15 STR loci of AmpFlSTR identifiler are shown, CSF1PO, D7S820, D8S1179, and D21S11). A heterozygous partial mole (**a**) harbors diandric heterozygous paternal alleles in addition to one maternal allele at every locus. Heterozygosity is evidenced by two distinct paternal alleles at some loci. A homozygous partial mole (**b**) contains diandric homozygous paternal alleles in addition to one maternal allele. Homozygosity is evidenced by one paternal allele with a duplicate copy number at all loci. The unique paternal alleles are indicated by an asterisk (Reproduced with permission from Hui P, 2011, Springer)

5.3.5.7 Non-Molar Mosaic Conceptions

Presence of an admixture of both androgenetic and biparental cell population within individual villi is reflected as paternal allelic excess (paternal allelic enrichment) with variable allelic ratios, often greater than 2:1 at informative STR loci.

5.3.5.8 Androgenetic/Biparental Mosaic Conceptions with a Non-molar Mosaic Component and a Molar Component

These are characterized by an admixture of p57-ve androgenetic villi representing CHM and villi with discordant p57 staining characteristic of non-molar mosaic conception, with each component being similar to the pure forms of these entities. Each component can be microdissected and individually genotyped with identical results as in the pure forms.

5.4 Algorithmic Approach for Diagnosis in Molar Gestation

Modern-day practice in the diagnosis of molar gestation recommends an algorithmic approach with indispensable use of ancillary techniques to facilitate categorization with reasonable confidence and avoid burden due to misclassification [18, 22, 24–26].

p57 immunohistochemical evaluation serves as a reasonable intermediary between histomorphological diagnosis and DNA genotyping. In most cases, the crucial subset of complete hydatidiform moles that require surveillance for persistent GTD can be confidently delineated from the rest by immunohistochemical evaluation of p57, whose interpretation is objective and reproducible in comparison to just histomorphology.

In a clinical setting where familial biparental complete hydatidiform mole is suspected, genetic analysis for relevant mutations is recommended in addition to DNA genotyping interpreted in the light of findings of p57 testing.

DNA genotyping is desirable in all p57+ve specimens, potentially partial hydatidiform moles as they confer a real, albeit low-risk rates for persistent GTD.

A diagnosis of a partial mole or non-molar gestation established on morphologic findings alone is negatively impacted by interobserver variability even among experts thereby reiterating the need to resort to an integrated approach of diagnosis including morphologic correlation, p57 immunohistochemistry, and DNA genotyping (Fig. 5.8).

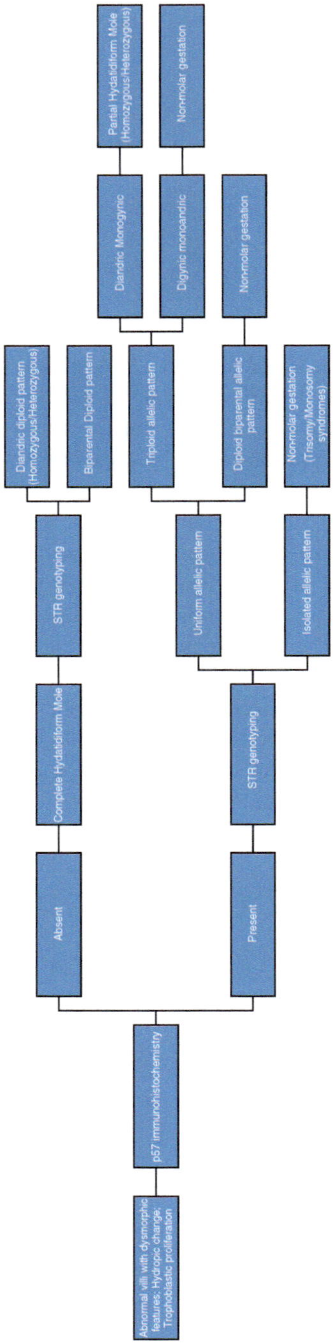

Fig. 5.8 An algorithmic approach for diagnosis of GTD

Disclaimer The authors of this chapter have no personal experience of utilizing these tests in routine practice and this chapter is written primarily based on understanding the nature of the disease, these tests and their utility in routine practice.

References

1. Vang R, Gupta M, Lee-Shu-Fune Wu AV, Yemelyanova RJK, Murphy KM, DeScipio C, et al. Diagnostic reproducibility of hydatidiform moles: ancillary techniques (p57 immunohistochemistry and molecular genotyping) improve morphologic diagnosis. Am J Surg Pathol. 2012;36(3):443.
2. Feltmate CM, Growdon WB, Wolfberg AJ, Goldstein DP, Genest DR, Chinchilla ME, et al. Clinical characteristics of persistent gestational trophoblastic neoplasia after partial hydatidiform molar pregnancy. J Reprod Med. 2006;51(11):902–6.
3. Berkowitz RS, Goldstein DP. Molar pregnancy. New Engl J Med. 2009;360(16):1639–45.
4. Hui P. Molecular diagnosis of gestational trophoblastic disease. Exp Rev Mol Diagn. 2010;10(8):1023–34.
5. Lipata F, Parkash V, Talmor M, Bell S, Chen S, Maric V, et al. Precise DNA genotyping diagnosis of hydatidiform mole. Obstet Gynecol. 2010;115(4):784–94.
6. Hayward BE, De Vos M, Talati N, Abdollahi MR, Taylor GR, Meyer E, et al. Genetic and epigenetic analysis of recurrent hydatidiform mole. Hum Mutat. 2009;30(5):E629–E39.
7. Van den Veyver I, Al-Hussaini T. Biparental hydatidiform moles: a maternal effect mutation affecting imprinting in the offspring. Hum Reprod Update 2006;12(3):233–42.
8. Hodges M, Rees H, Seckl M, Newlands E, Fisher R. Genetic refinement and physical mapping of a biparental complete hydatidiform mole locus on chromosome 19q13.4. J Med Genet. 2003;40(8):e95.
9. Judson H, Hayward BE, Sheridan E, Bonthron DT. A global disorder of imprinting in the human female germ line. Nature. 2002;416(6880):539–42.
10. Kou YC, Shao L, Peng HH, Rosetta R, del Gaudio D, Wagner AF, et al. A recurrent intragenic genomic duplication, other novel mutations in NLRP7 and imprinting defects in recurrent biparental hydatidiform moles. MHR Basic Sci Reprod Med. 2007;14(1):33–40.
11. Mahadevan S, Wen S, Wan Y-W, Peng H-H, Otta S, Liu Z, et al. NLRP7 affects trophoblast lineage differentiation, binds to overexpressed YY1 and alters CpG methylation. Hum Mol Genet. 2013;23(3):706–16.
12. Redline RW, Hassold T, Zaragoza MV. Prevalence of the partial molar phenotype in triploidy of maternal and paternal origin. Hum Pathol. 1998;29(5):505–11.
13. Uchida IA, Freeman VC. Triploidy and chromosomes. Am J Obstet Gynecol. 1985;151(1):65–9.
14. Ronnett BM. Hydatidiform moles: ancillary techniques to refine diagnosis. Arch Pathol Lab Med. 2018;142(12):1485–502.
15. Hoffner L, Dunn J, Esposito N, Macpherson T, Surti U. P57KIP2 immunostaining and molecular cytogenetics: combined approach aids in diagnosis of morphologically challenging cases with molar phenotype and in detecting androgenetic cell lines in mosaic/chimeric conceptions. Hum Pathol. 2008;39(1):63–72.
16. Hoffner L, Parks WT, Swerdlow SH, Carson JC, Surti U. Simultaneous detection of imprinted gene expression (p57 (KIP2)) and molecular cytogenetics (FICTION) in the evaluation of molar pregnancies. J Reprod Med. 2010;55(5–6):219–28.
17. Lewis GH, DeScipio C, Murphy KM, Haley L, Beierl K, Mosier S, et al. Characterization of androgenetic/biparental mosaic/chimeric conceptions, including those with a molar component: morphology, p57 immnohistochemistry, molecular genotyping, and risk of persistent gestational trophoblastic disease. Int J Gynecol Pathol. 2013;32(2):199–214.

18. Ronnett BM, DeScipio C, Murphy KM. Hydatidiform moles: ancillary techniques to refine diagnosis. Int J Gynecol Pathol. 2011;30(2):101–16.
19. McConnell TG, Norris-Kirby A, Hagenkord JM, Ronnett BM, Murphy KM. Complete hydatidiform mole with retained maternal chromosomes 6 and 11. Am J Surg Pathol. 2009;33(9):1409–15.
20. Fisher RA, Nucci MR, Thaker HM, Weremowicz S, Genest DR, Castrillon DH. Complete hydatidiform mole retaining a chromosome 11 of maternal origin: molecular genetic analysis of a case. Mod Pathol. 2004;17(9):1155.
21. DeScipio C, Haley L, Beierl K, Pandit AP, Murphy KM, Ronnett BM. Diandric triploid hydatidiform mole with loss of maternal chromosome 11. Am J Surg Pathol. 2011;35(10):1586–91.
22. Banet N, DeScipio C, Murphy KM, Beierl K, Adams E, Vang R, et al. Characteristics of hydatidiform moles: analysis of a prospective series with p57 immunohistochemistry and molecular genotyping. Mod Pathol. 2014;27(2):238.
23. Chiang S, Fazlollahi L, Nguyen A, Betensky RA, Roberts DJ, Iafrate AJ. Diagnosis of hydatidiform moles by polymorphic deletion probe fluorescence in situ hybridization. J Mol Diagn. 2011;13(4):406–15.
24. McConnell TG, Murphy KM, Hafez M, Vang R, Ronnett BM. Diagnosis and subclassification of hydatidiform moles using p57 immunohistochemistry and molecular genotyping: validation and prospective analysis in routine and consultation practice settings with development of an algorithmic approach. Am J Surg Pathol. 2009;33(6):805–17.
25. Murphy KM, Ronnett BM. Molecular analysis of hydatidiform moles: utilizing p57 immunohistochemistry and molecular genotyping to refine morphologic diagnosis. AJSP Rev Rep. 2010;15(4):126–34.
26. Buza N, Hui P. Immunohistochemistry and other ancillary techniques in the diagnosis of gestational trophoblastic diseases. Semin Diagn Pathol. 2014;31(3):223–32.

Imaging in Gestational Trophoblastic Disease and Implication of Uterine Artery Doppler Study

6

Goldwin H. Cecil, Anuradha Chandramohan, and Abraham Peedicayil

6.1 Introduction

Gestational trophoblastic disease (GTD) includes a broad spectrum of clinical diseases that arise from placental tissue and range from benign to malignant conditions. Around 15–20% of complete hydatidiform moles (CHM) and 0.5% of partial hydatidiform moles (PHM) advance to invasive mole, choriocarcinoma, placental site trophoblastic tumor (PSTT), and epithelioid trophoblastic tumor (ETT). The latter are collectively called gestational trophoblastic neoplasms (GTN) [1]. Early clinical suspicion and accurate diagnosis will have a great impact on reducing the morbidity in these patients. Though most of the persistent trophoblastic diseases follow benign hydatidiform moles, GTN can also occur after miscarriages, ectopic pregnancies, and even normal pregnancies. Prompt diagnosis will preserve fertility, reduce the use of chemotherapy, and improve outcomes. The role of imaging in the management of gestational trophoblastic diseases is crucial to accomplish this goal.

There are geographic variations in the incidence of GTD with the highest incidence reported in South East Asia [2]. Although there may be true variations in incidence, some of the variability may be due to differences in how the numerator and the denominator are arrived at. The predisposing factors for the increased incidence include the extremes of ages, i.e., <20 years and > 40 years and previous molar pregnancy [3]. GTN is known to arise from CHM, PHM, miscarriages, or even term delivery. The incidence of choriocarcinoma after a term delivery is 1/50,000 [4].

G. H. Cecil · A. Chandramohan (✉)
Department of Radiology, Christian Medical College, Vellore, India
e-mail: anuradha.chandramohan@cmcvellore.ac.in

A. Peedicayil
Department of Gynaecologic Oncology, Christian Medical College and Hospital, Vellore, India
e-mail: abraham@cmcvellore.ac.in

B. Nayak, U. Singh (eds.), *Gestational Trophoblastic Disease*,
https://doi.org/10.1007/978-981-33-4878-3_6

Vaginal bleeding in early pregnancy should raise the suspicion of a molar pregnancy apart from ectopic pregnancy and some form of abortion. Along with clinical examination, quantitative assessment of the β-hCG levels and ultrasonography play a valuable role in the early diagnosis of a hydatidiform mole. Color Doppler study and subsequent follow-up of hCG values will help in diagnosing post-molar sequelae. CT of the chest abdomen and pelvis and MRI of the pelvis and brain have vital roles in the accurate staging and prognostication of GTN, the diagnosis of which is made mainly on the basis of rise or plateau of serum hCG values.

6.2 Pathology

Almost 95% of CHM have a 46 XX karyotype when an abnormal ovum devoid of maternal chromosomes is fertilized by one or more haploid sperm in an attempt at parthenogenesis. If a single sperm is involved, the paternal chromosomes duplicate to establish a diploid karyotype. The gross specimen has an appearance like a bunch of grapes, due to edematous villi formed from cytotrophoblasts and syncytiotrophoblasts [5].

Majority of PHMs are triploid karyotypes when a single haploid ovum is fertilized by two sperms. In PHM, there is less villous edema and there is usually an abnormal embryo that rarely survives beyond the second trimester. Diagnosis of PHM is often missed since the uterine size may be near normal, imaging findings are usually subtle and the β-hCG levels may not be significantly increased. Molecular genotyping using either polymorphic STR analysis or alternatively analysis by whole genome SNP microarray can be used to differentiate a CHM from a PHM and non-molar abortions.

Persistent elevation of β-hCG values after evacuation of a CHM or a PHM is the hallmark of GTN. Invasive mole is characterized by varying degrees of myometrial invasion. Choriocarcinoma is the most aggressive form of GTN and has necrotic and hemorrhagic components. Histologically, choriocarcinomas resemble an implanting blastocyst with no formed chorionic villi. Presentation can be varied and can even present years after conception or may occur de novo in the uterus. It is angio-invasive and hematogenous hypervascular metastasis most commonly to lungs, liver, brain, and vagina [6].

Placental site trophoblastic tumor (PSTT) and epithelioid trophoblastic tumor (ETT) are rare forms of GTN, which share many similarities. They arise in the placental implantation site from the intermediate trophoblasts in young women of reproductive age group following a pregnancy. Both these tumors occur more commonly following normal delivery, yet can occur following CHM, PHM, and miscarriages. They are slow-growing tumors with propensity for local invasion and lymph node metastases [7]. Serum hCG levels are not very high in these patients and they respond poorly to chemotherapy. Thus, surgery remains the main treatment of choice [8].

Table 6.1 FIGO staging (2006) of gestational trophoblastic neoplasms

Stage	Tumor extent
Stage I	Tumor confined to the uterus
Stage II	Tumor extends beyond the uterus, limited to the genital structures
Stage III	Tumor extends to the lungs, with or without known genital tract involvement
Stage IV	Tumor involves all other metastatic sites

Table 6.2 Revised FIGO prognostic scoring 2006

FIGO score	0	1	2	4
Age (years)	<40	≥40	–	–
Antecedent pregnancy	Mole	Abortion	Term	–
Interval months from the index pregnancy	<4 months	4–6 months	6–12 months	>1 year
Pretreatment hCG (mIU/ml)	<1000	1000–10,000	10,000- 1,00,000	>1,00,000
Largest tumor size including uterus (cm)	<3	3–5	>5	–
Site of metastases	Lung	Spleen, kidney	Gastrointestinal	Brain, liver
Number of metastasis	–	1–4	5–8	>8
Previously failed chemotherapy	–	–	Single drug	Two or more drugs

(Prognostic scoring for GTN based on clinical features, total serum β-hCG, and chest X-ray)

6.3 Staging

The FIGO staging is an anatomical one that does not correlate very well with biological behavior and prognosis. The WHO/FIGO prognostic scoring system should be used along with the anatomical staging to make management decisions. These are given in Tables 6.1 and 6.2.

6.4 Role of Imaging in the Management of GTD

Ultrasonography and color Doppler study are the imaging modalities of choice in the initial evaluation and diagnosis of GTD. Cross-sectional imaging methods such as contrast-enhanced CT, MRI, and PET-CT have important roles in the staging and surveillance of patients with GTNGTN. These tests can be ordered when specific indications arise and is going to decide the management protocol.

6.5 Ultrasonography

Ultrasound of pelvis is the first radiological investigation of choice in the evaluation of women with vaginal bleeding during pregnancy. One cannot emphasize the role of ultrasound and doppler in the diagnosis of GTD. With improved imaging, diagnosis is now made much earlier than in the past.

The most common finding in a woman with CHM is an enlarged uterus with echogenic endometrial contents [9]. Though missed abortion may have similar findings, presence of elevated β-hCG must raise suspicion of CHM. The characteristic image of a CHM on ultrasound is the "snow-storm" in A-mode or "honeycomb" or "cluster of grapes" appearance in B-mode. Higher resolution of transvaginal ultrasound will allow better visualization of the interface between the uterine myometrium and the trophoblastic tissue and helps with identifying myometrial invasion. Multiple anechoic vesicles of varying sizes (ranging between 1 and 30 mm) formed from hydropic chorionic villi give the typical appearance (Figs. 6.1 and 6.2) on

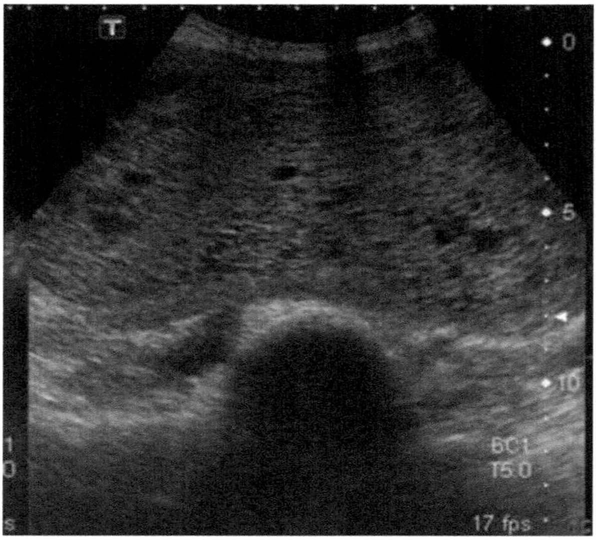

Fig. 6.1 Ultrasound image of the complete hydatiform mole showing echogenic mass and multiple cystic spaces in an enlarged uterus

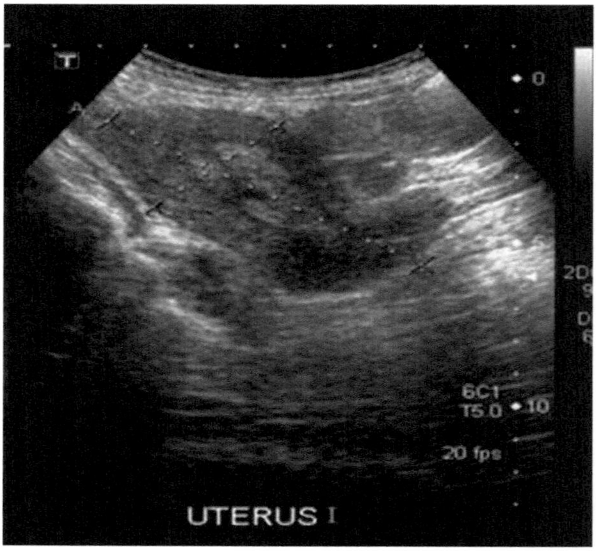

Fig. 6.2 Ultrasonography of a patient with invasive mole showing invasion into the anterior myometrium where there is loss of smooth interface between the echogenic mass and the myometrium

B-mode ultrasound [10]. In addition, large irregular cystic spaces from cystic degeneration may be seen within the endometrial mass. These findings become obvious even in the transabdominal ultrasound by the second trimester due to large uterine size and increase in the size and the number of the vesicles. Confirmation of myometrial invasion or excluding the same is crucial prior to suction evacuation of the uterus since the invasive component cannot be removed with evacuation [11] and these patients are likely to have persistent disease. Fetal parts or the fetus is typically absent in CHM unless rarely when CHM coexists with a diploid twin. About 20% of CHM have theca lutein cysts from ovarian hyperstimulation [12].

In PHM, there is thickened placenta with anechoic cystic spaces much fewer in number when compared to CHM [13]. This is usually associated with the presence of oval gestational sac, amniotic membrane, and a nonviable or incompletely formed embryo [14]. Naumoff et al. established criteria for diagnosing PHM stating that the placenta should be enlarged with numerous anechoic spaces, with a gestational sac and retarded growth of the fetus [15].

Table 6.3 summarizes the ultrasound imaging features of CHM and PHM. Differentiating CHM from PHM has prognostic significance due to the

Table 6.3 Ultrasound and Doppler features of CHM, PHM, incomplete abortion, and GTN

Feature	CHM	PHM	Incomplete abortion	GTN
Uterine size	Larger than appropriate for dates	Smaller than appropriate for dates	Smaller than appropriate for dates	Variable, usually enlarged uterus
Placental size	Normal	Enlarged and thickened	Normal	Absent
Placental architecture	Normal	Multiple anechoic cysts in the placenta	Normal	Absent
Fetal tissue	Absent	Present, usually non-viable	Present, non-viability is a rule	Absent
USG pattern	Snowstorm appearance	Swiss cheese appearance	Hyperechoic contents in the endometrial cavity	Heterogeneous echogenic mass. Loss of endometrium myometrium interface
Theca lutein cysts	Common	Less common	Rare	Common
Doppler color flow	Increased uterine vasculature, limited to the cystic vascular spaces in the endometrium	Increased uterine vasculature, limited to the cystic vascular spaces in the endometrium	Multiple feeding vessels around the hyperechoic contents	Increased vasculature with abnormal arteriovenous malformations. Vascular spaces extend into the myometrium
Resistivity index (RI)	Lower limit of normal (0.55)	Lower limit of normal (0.55)	Normal (0.66)	Low resistance flow (0.28)

differences in the rates of developing GTN in these conditions. While 15–20% of CHM progress to GTN, only 0.5% of PHM develop GTN. Though the differences between the ultrasound findings between these two entities have been well described, less than 50% of GTD are detected on routine ultrasound with obviously better detection rates for CHM (58–95%) when compared to PHM (17–29%) [16–18]. The overall sensitivity, specificity, PPV, and NPV of ultrasound for diagnosing any form of gestational trophoblastic disease is 44, 77, 88, and 23%, respectively [16]. Thus, the need for histopathological analysis of the products of conception of all nonviable pregnancies becomes essential.

The purpose of ultrasound in patients with clinically suspected GTN due to persistently elevated β-hCG following suction evacuation of molar pregnancy is to exclude normal intrauterine pregnancy, to measure the size of the mass and the uterus and, to assess the extent of local spread of disease [19]. The imaging features of GTN are by themselves nonspecific and may appear as hypoechoic or hyperechoic heterogeneous endometrial mass due to hemorrhage and necrosis. Following the diagnosis of GTD, ultrasound of the whole abdomen in GTN is usually the initial imaging procedure.

6.6 Color Doppler Study

Color Doppler study has the capability of noninvasively demonstrating the same findings as the pelvic arteriogram and has been shown to be of value in the management of GTN.

6.6.1 Doppler in Differentiating CHM and PHM

In clinical practice, uterine artery Doppler indices cannot be used to differentiate between CHM and PHM. However, Doppler indices are useful for identifying CHM coexisting with a normal fetus. Uterine artery RI (UA-RI) in normal pregnancy is significantly higher (mean RI = 0.66 ± 0.05) than the UA-RI in CHM (mean RI = 0.56 ± 0.04) and PHM (mean RI = 0.55 ± 0.06) [20].

6.6.2 Doppler in the Prediction of GTN and Chemoresistance

Color Doppler studies have potential roles in the prediction of GTN both before and following the evacuation of molar pregnancy. Lower UA Doppler indices were associated with the development of GTN (mean Resistive Index (RI) = 0.29) when compared to those who had spontaneous remission (mean RI = 0.46) [21, 22]. Presence of myometrial and endometrial nodules or masses showing hypervascularity 3 weeks after evacuation of the molar pregnancy highly correlated with the development of GTN. However, they are late findings. Doppler flow velocimetry can potentially identify disease early much before ultrasound findings can be seen.

While the negative predictive value of a normal Doppler study was 100% for development of GTN, the positive predictive value of abnormal Doppler findings 6 weeks following evacuation was 67% for residual local disease [24]. Of all the Doppler indices, Pulsatility Index (PI) was found to have the strongest predictor of developing GTN pre and post evacuation of CHM. PI is a parameter that assesses the pulsatility of the blood flow and it is given as the difference between the maximum and minimal flow velocity normalized to the time-averaged velocity. The formula for calculating PI is (peak systolic velocity (PSV)—end diastolic velocity (EDV))/time-averaged velocity (TAV). On the other hand resistive index (RI) is a measure of resistance to blood flow caused by microvascular bed, which is distal to the index vessel. The formula for calculated RI is (PSV—EDV)/PSV.

A PI value of </=1.3 pre-evacuation predicted the development of GTN with 77% sensitivity and 87% specificity. A cutoff value of PI</=1.7 post evacuation predicted the development of GTN with 79% sensitivity and 86% specificity [23]. PI < 1.1 is associated with chemoresistance to methotrexate and such low PI is an indirect evidence of increased tumor neovascularization and arteriovenous shunting [24].

In summary, uterine artery Doppler indices significantly increase in patients with spontaneous remission of molar pregnancy while they remained low in patients who are at risk of developing GTN. PI is the most useful parameter available to study the risk of developing GTN pre and post evaluation of molar pregnancy. Low PI value of <1.1 can predict resistance to methotrexate.

Figure 6.3 shows the Ultrasound—Color Doppler appearance of choriocarcinoma and the high-velocity low-resistance flow in the tumor vessels. Also demonstrated are the right and left uterine artery velocimetry values and spectral trace in these vessels.

6.7 Computed Tomography and MRI

CT has little role in the primary diagnosis of GTN. When identified CT can show a hypervascular uterine mass in patients with choriocarcinoma (Fig. 6.4) with parametrial infiltration (Fig. 6.5). Contrast-enhanced CT of the thorax, abdomen, and pelvis is useful for staging of proven GTN.

FIGO recommends plain chest radiograph for evaluation of metastases to the lungs. The importance of solitary metastases is yet to be analyzed completely. The clinical outcomes related to the number of metastases are also not clear. But it is common for CT to detect more lesions in the lungs compared to plain chest radiographs. However, small lesions seen only on CT are not used in the prognostic scoring. CT thorax can be advised if patient is symptomatic to rule out pulmonary thromboembolism. In high-risk patients, a CT thorax is recommended as plain film does not pick up about 41% of the lung metastases (Fig. 6.6). Liver metastases occur much later in the disease process and have poor prognosis. Liver metastases are hypervascular and these lesions should not be biopsied due to risk of life-threatening hemorrhage.

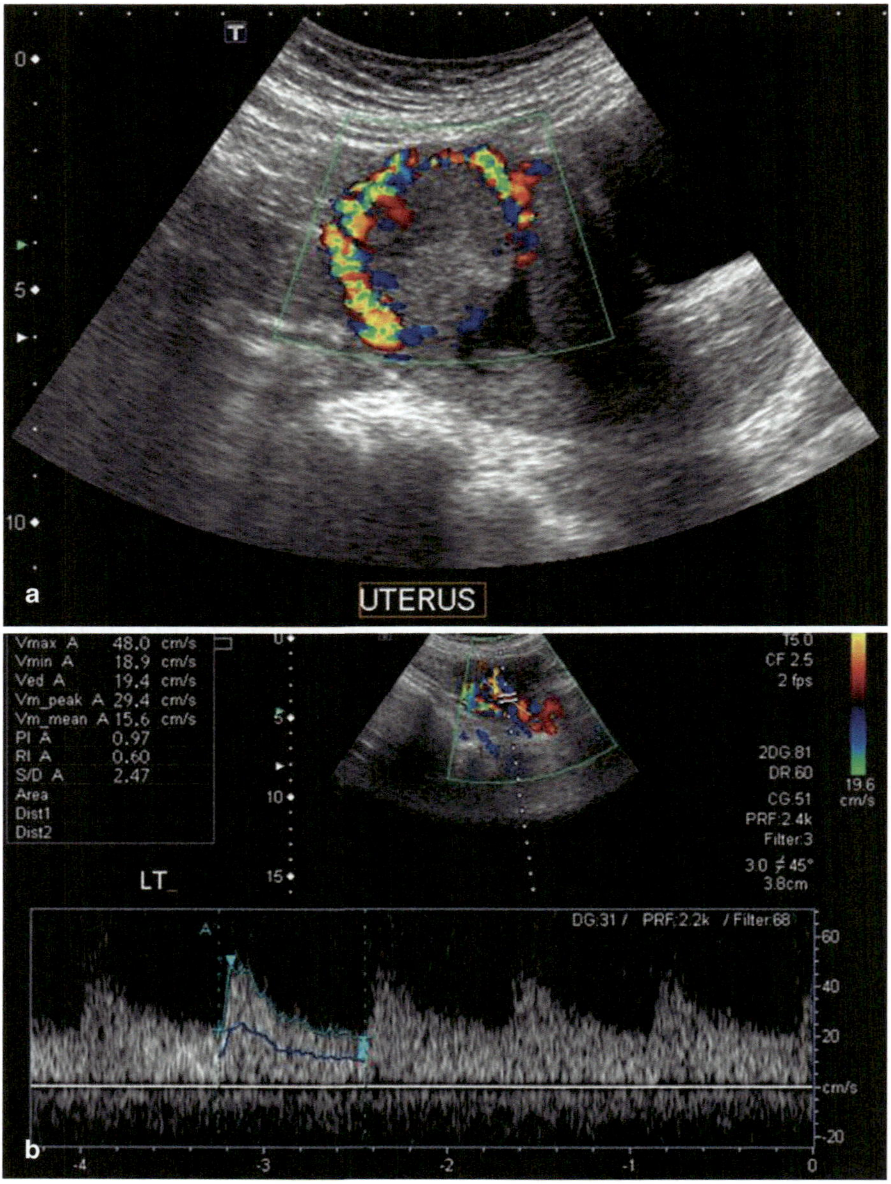

Fig. 6.3 Color Doppler image (**a**) and Doppler flow velocimetry in choriocarcinoma in the left uterine artery (**b**). Notice the low pulsatility index (PI) and resistive index (RI)

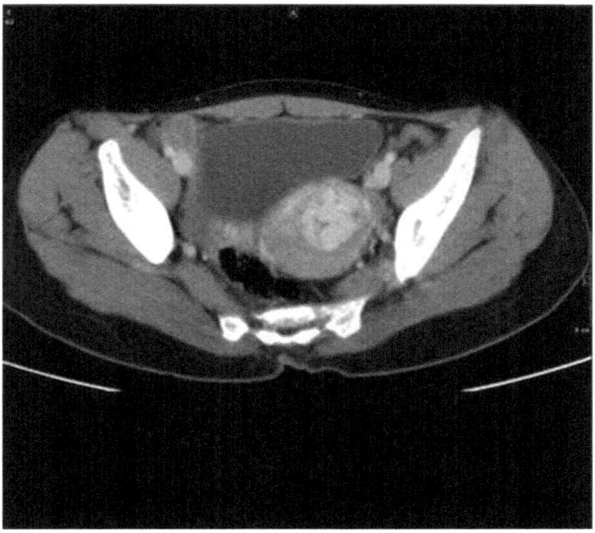

Fig. 6.4 CT abdomen showing enhancing mass in the uterus with possible myometrial invasion

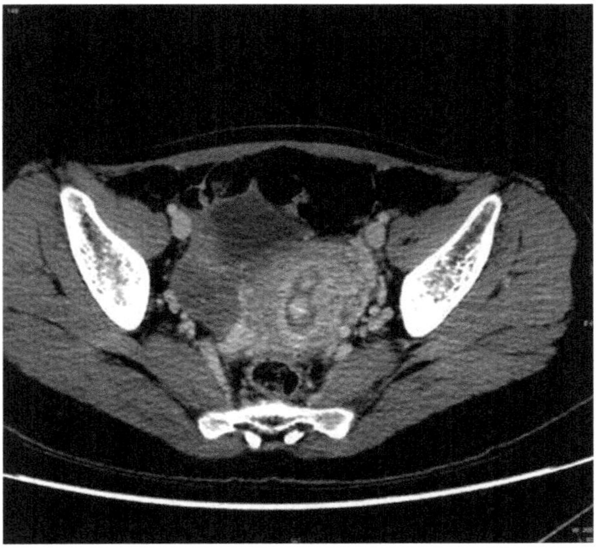

Fig. 6.5 CT Abdomen images of a patient with choriocarcinoma showing extension into the parametrium with the avid enhancement of the tumor

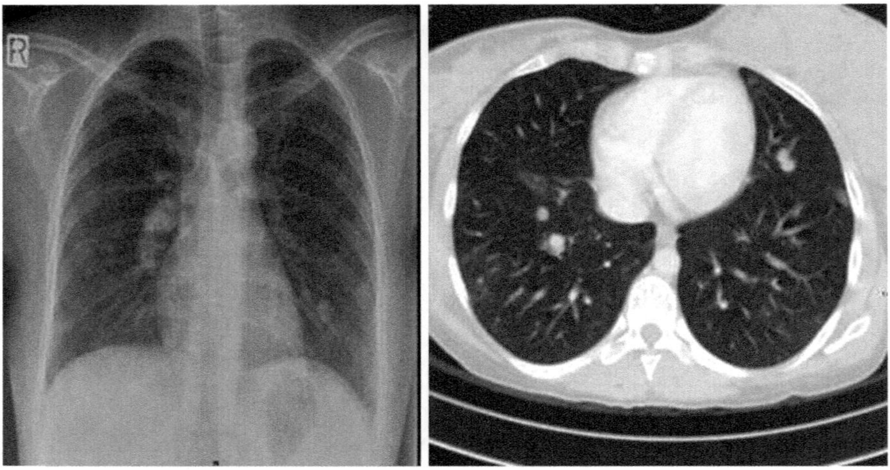

Fig. 6.6 Plain chest radiograph and CT thorax in lung window of a patient with choriocarcinoma showing multiple pulmonary metastases on CT

Central nervous system involvement has been noted in ~15% of the patients with metastatic disease. Patients with lung metastases are at increased risk of CNS spread. MRI of the brain is the investigation of choice for diagnosing brain metastases and for their follow up. Also, 85% of brain metastases occur in non-molar choriocarcinomas who have 20% risk of brain metastases. Thus, the importance of routinely imaging the brain in these patients [25]. On the other hand, the prevalence of brain metastases is extremely low in patients with post-molar choriocarcinomas.

MRI pelvis has a role in the local staging of disease in the pelvis. Metastases to the vagina are due to direct extension of primary uterine lesion and can occur in 30% of patients. MRI pelvis is the investigation of choice for these patients. Other regions involving metastases from GTD include the kidney, gastrointestinal tract, and the skin [26].

6.8 Digital Angiography and Intervention

Arteriovenous malformations (AVM) are a part of the normal pathogenesis of gestational trophoblastic neoplasms where there is direct communication between the arteries and the veins without an intervening capillary bed. Though most of them resolve after treatment for GTD, 10–15% of AVMs tend to persist even after a complete cure of GTD. Of these AVMs only ~2% of them may require treatment due to refractory vaginal bleeding [27, 28].

Color Doppler studies can be used for identifying AVMs, flow aneurysms, and arterio-venous fistulas, which show high-velocity low-resistance flow patterns with severe aliasing (misidentification of signals; see Fig. 6.7). Angiography shows a

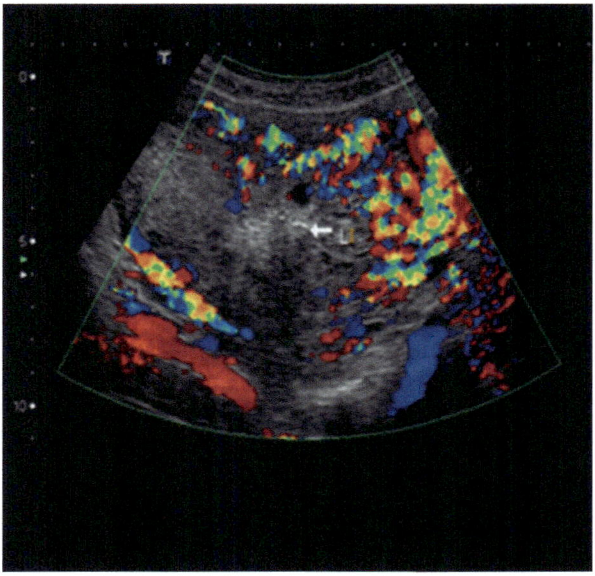

Fig. 6.7 Color Doppler study arteriovenous malformation in a patient with invasive mole recurrence, which is seen as a tangle of vessels in the uterus with color aliasing due to high flow

tangle of abnormal vessels at the nidus of the AVM with early venous filling. Super selective catheterization of the AVM with liquid embolization with glue or coil embolization may be performed to treat AVMs that present with bleed.

6.9 Conclusion and Key Points

Imaging plays a central role in the diagnosis, management, and the surveillance of gestational trophoblastic diseases.

- Ultrasound is the first imaging investigation of choice in the evaluation of bleeding during pregnancy.
- In patients with elevated β-hCG following evacuation of molar pregnancy, the main role of ultrasound is to exclude normal pregnancy.
- Measuring the size of the mass and the size of the uterus on ultrasound has prognostic significance.
- Doppler indices such as pulsatility index are useful in both diagnosing GTN and in predicting chemoresistance.
- In non-molar choriocarcinoma, staging evaluation should include CT of the thorax, abdomen, and pelvis (CT-TAP).
- In molar choriocarcinoma, CT abdomen pelvis and MR brain can be selectively done in patients with lung metastases.
- Symptomatic patients with AVMs following GTD can be treated with angio-embolization.

References

1. Altieri A, Franceschi S, Ferlay J, Smith J, La Vecchia C. Epidemiology and aetiology of gestational trophoblastic diseases. Lancet Oncol. 2003;4(11):670–8.
2. Ho HN, Gill TJ, Klionsky B, Ouyang PC, Hsieh CY, Seski J, et al. Differences between white and Chinese populations in human leukocyte antigen sharing and gestational trophoblastic tumors. Am J Obstet Gynecol. 1989;161(4):942–8.
3. Sebire NJ, Fisher RA, Foskett M, Rees H, Seckl MJ, Newlands ES. Risk of recurrent hydatidiform mole and subsequent pregnancy outcome following complete or partial hydatidiform molar pregnancy. BJOG Int J Obstet Gynaecol. 2003;110(1):22–6.
4. Seckl MJ, Fisher RA, Salerno G, Rees H, Paradinas FJ, Foskett M, et al. Choriocarcinoma and partial hydatidiform moles. Lancet Lond Engl. 2000;356(9223):36–9.
5. Allen SD, Lim AK, Seckl MJ, Blunt DM, Mitchell AW. Radiology of gestational trophoblastic neoplasia. Clin Radiol. 2006;61(4):301–13.
6. Ng TY, Wong LC. Diagnosis and management of gestational trophoblastic neoplasia. Best Pract Res Clin Obstet Gynaecol. 2003;17(6):893–903.
7. Feltmate CM, Genest DR, Wise L, Bernstein MR, Goldstein DP, Berkowitz RS. Placental site trophoblastic tumor: a 17-year experience at the New England trophoblastic disease center. Gynecol Oncol. 2001;82(3):415–9.
8. Hunter V, Raymond E, Christensen C, Olt G, Soper J, Hammond C. Efficacy of the metastatic survey in the staging of gestational trophoblastic disease. Cancer. 1990;65(7):1647–50.
9. DeBaz BP, Lewis TJ. Imaging of gestational trophoblastic disease. Semin Oncol. 1995;22(2):130–41.
10. Dehner LP. Gestational and nongestational trophoblastic neoplasia: a historic and pathobiologic survey. Am J Surg Pathol. 1980;4(1):43–58.
11. Green CL, Angtuaco TL, Shah HR, Parmley TH. Gestational trophoblastic disease: a spectrum of radiologic diagnosis. Radiogr Rev Publ Radiol Soc N Am Inc. 1996;16(6):1371–84.
12. Hou J-L, Wan X-R, Xiang Y, Qi Q-W, Yang X-Y. Changes of clinical features in hydatidiform mole: analysis of 113 cases. J Reprod Med. 2008;53(8):629–33.
13. Sonographic and Doppler imaging in the diagnosis and treatment of gestational trophoblastic disease: a 12-year experience. PubMed—NCBI [Internet]. [cited 2019 Feb 11]. Retrieved from: https://www.ncbi.nlm.nih.gov/pubmed/15615924
14. Szulman AE, Surti U. The syndromes of hydatidiform mole. II. Morphologic evolution of the complete and partial mole. Am J Obstet Gynecol. 1978;132(1):20–7.
15. Ultrasonography of partial hydatidiform mole. | Radiology [Internet]. [cited 2019 Feb 11]. Retrieved from: https://pubs.rsna.org/doi/10.1148/radiology.140.2.7255725.
16. Fowler DJ, Lindsay I, Seckl MJ, Sebire NJ. Routine pre-evacuation ultrasound diagnosis of hydatidiform mole: experience of more than 1000 cases from a regional referral center. Ultrasound Obstet Gynecol Off J Int Soc Ultrasound Obstet Gynecol. 2006;27(1):56–60.
17. Kirk E, Papageorghiou AT, Condous G, Bottomley C, Bourne T. The accuracy of first trimester ultrasound in the diagnosis of hydatidiform mole. Ultrasound Obstet Gynecol Off J Int Soc Ultrasound Obstet Gynecol. 2007;29(1):70–5.
18. Sebire NJ, Rees H, Paradinas F, Seckl M, Newlands E. The diagnostic implications of routine ultrasound examination in histologically confirmed early molar pregnancies. Ultrasound Obstet Gynecol Off J Int Soc Ultrasound Obstet Gynecol. 2001;18(6):662–5.
19. Mangili G, Lorusso D, Brown J, Pfisterer J, Massuger L, Vaughan M, et al. Trophoblastic disease review for diagnosis and management: a joint report from the International Society for the Study of trophoblastic disease, European organisation for the treatment of trophoblastic disease, and the Gynecologic cancer InterGroup. Int J Gynecol Cancer Off J Int Gynecol Cancer Soc. 2014;24(9 Suppl 3):S109–16.
20. Zhou Q, Lei X-Y, Xie Q, Cardoza JD. Sonographic and Doppler imaging in the diagnosis and treatment of gestational trophoblastic disease: a 12-year experience. J Ultrasound Med Off J Am Inst Ultrasound Med. 2005;24(1):15–24.

21. Gungor T, Ekin M, Dumanli H, Gokmen O. Color Doppler ultrasonography in the earlier differentiation of benign molehydatidiforms from malignant gestational trophoblastic disease. Acta Obstet Gynecol Scand. 1998;77(8):860–2.
22. Yalcin OT, Ozalp SS, Tanir HM. Assessment of gestational trophoblastic disease by Doppler ultrasonography. Eur J Obstet Gynecol Reprod Biol. 2002;103(1):83–7.
23. Asmar FTC, Braga-Neto AR, de Rezende-Filho J, Villas-Boas JMS, Charry RC, Maesta I, et al. Uterine artery Doppler flow velocimetry parameters for predicting gestational trophoblastic neoplasia after complete hydatidiform mole, a prospective cohort study. Clinics. 2017;72(5):284–8.
24. Agarwal R, Harding V, Short D, Fisher RA, Sebire NJ, Harvey R, et al. Uterine artery pulsatility index: a predictor of methotrexate resistance in gestational trophoblastic neoplasia. Br J Cancer. 2012;106(6):1089–94.
25. Savage P, Kelpanides I, Tuthill M, Short D, Seckl MJ. Brain metastases in gestational trophoblast neoplasia: an update on incidence, management and outcome. Gynecol Oncol. 2015;137(1):73–6.
26. May T, Goldstein DP, Berkowitz RS. Current chemotherapeutic management of patients with gestational trophoblastic neoplasia. Chemother Res Pract. 2011;2011:806256.
27. Touhami O, Gregoire J, Noel P, Trinh XB, Plante M. Uterine arteriovenous malformations following gestational trophoblastic neoplasia: a systematic review. Eur J Obstet Gynecol Reprod Biol. 2014;181:54–9.
28. Embolization of bleeding residual uterine vascular malformations in patients with treated gestational trophoblastic tumors. PubMed – NCBI [Internet]. [cited 2019 Feb 25]. Retrieved from: https://www.ncbi.nlm.nih.gov/pubmed/11867779

Hydatidiform Mole with Coexisting Live Foetus: Management Guidelines

7

Uma Singh, Manju Lata Verma, and Sabuhi Qureshi

Hydatidiform mole with coexisting live foetus presents a management enigma. It can happen either as a consequence of dizygotic twin gestation in which complete hydatidiform mole is associated with coexisting live foetus (CHMCF) or partial mole with live foetus. Differentiation between these two entities is important because treatment for partial mole with live foetus is termination of pregnancy while in cases with CHMCF, pregnancy can be continued but only under strict maternal and foetal surveillance.

7.1 Diagnosis

On ultrasound, presence of grape-like vesicles or snow storm appearance without foetal structures suggests diagnosis of a complete mole. If there is a placenta with molar changes, in addition to foetus with cardiac activity, diagnosis of partial mole with live foetus is made. However, diagnosis of CHMCF is made, if there is a presence of diamniotic dichorionic twin gestation with one amniotic sac having normal placenta with live foetus and one sac is having complete mole. For precise diagnosis of partial and complete mole, genotyping at molecular level is required. Amniocentesis or chorionic villus sampling can be done for segregation analysis of parental and placental alleles [1].

U. Singh (✉) · M. L. Verma
KG Medical University, Lucknow, India

S. Qureshi
Super Speciality Cancer Institute, Lucknow, India

B. Nayak, U. Singh (eds.), *Gestational Trophoblastic Disease*,
https://doi.org/10.1007/978-981-33-4878-3_7

7.2 Partial Hydatidiform Mole with Live Foetus

Karyotype will be triploid in partial mole and both parental (maternal and paternal) genes will be present while in complete mole, karyotype will be diploid and all the genes will be from paternal origin [2]. If dispermic fertilization occurs, triploidy in partial mole consists of one maternal and two paternal haploid sets. In this situation, triploid foetus with large placenta is found. Placenta is large because of the presence of hydropic villi that are dispersed with normal chorionic villi. Very early demise of foetus occurs in this type of fertilization. If digynic fertilization occurs, growth restriction is a prominent feature in foetus and placenta is small as villi exhibit very minimal hydropic changes. There are very rare chances of having live birth in these pregnancies but in case it continues, it ultimately culminates in neonatal death.

Partial mole with triploid foetus is lethal for foetus and usually results in spontaneous abortion, so treatment is termination of pregnancy. However, maternal complications in terms of preeclampsia and placental trophoblastic disease are not higher when compared to complete molar pregnancy [1]. The chances of development of persistent GTD or malignant complication in partial mole is 0.5%.

Possibility of placental mesenchymal dysplasia (PMD) should always be ruled out in which a similar ultrasound picture is found. This includes placentomegaly with cystic changes in placenta. Differentiation between the two entities is must as management and outcome differ. PMD with live foetus pregnancies should not be terminated. However, the risk of intrauterine growth restriction, preterm birth, and stillbirth need to be explained to the couple. With presence of normal foetus on ultrasound and diploid karyotype, low-velocity colour flow within the cystic placental mass on colour Doppler, the possibility of PMD should be considered. Mesenchymal stem villous hyperplasia on histopathology is diagnostic for PMD.

7.3 Complete Hydatidiform Mole with Coexisting Live Foetus (CHMCF)

Complete hydatidiform mole with coexisting live foetus is an uncommon presentation [3] and its occurrence in literature is found to be 1 in 22,000 to 1 in 100,000 [4]. Pregnancies with coexisting live foetus with complete mole can be continued with strict foetomaternal surveillance. Since these foetuses are karyotypically normal, if these pregnancies pass beyond 32 weeks of gestation, chances of survival are as high as 25–40% [5, 6]. However, these patients are more prone to complications in terms of preeclampsia, antepartum haemorrhage, and placental trophoblastic disease and choriocarcinoma [7, 8].

7.4 Management Guidelines

Since pregnancies with complete mole with coexisting live foetus are not common and at very high risk for complications a proper, well-informed written consent is needed before couple agrees to continue with pregnancy.

Arrangement should be made for proper and timely referral to a tertiary care centre if any complication arises.

Antepartum haemorrhage is the most common complication occurring in 60% of pregnancies. Continuation or termination depends upon amount of blood loss and foetomaternal condition. The increased incidence of vaginal bleeding in these pregnancies may be because of low implantation of these molar tissues [9].

These pregnancies should be strictly monitored for development of preeclampsia. Risk of developing this complication is 20%. Management will depend upon the gestation at which preeclampsia arises and also upon its severity. This is an independent predictor of poor infant survival if severe preeclampsia occurs at early gestational age [10].

Risk of developing hyperemesis gravidarum is as high as in 7% of cases and should be managed carefully.

These pregnant patients also have a 15% chance of developing hyperthyroidism. Sometimes pregnancy needs to be terminated for maternal indication.

Arrangement of senior paediatrician and NICU care is a must while managing these pregnancies as most of them need to be terminated at preterm gestation in presence of maternal complications.

In post-partum period, these patients have to be followed for post molar GTN. Risk of developing choriocarcinoma is 15–20%. The higher is the initial level of beta HCG; the more is the chance of developing choriocarcinoma. Niemann et al. [11] showed in their study that although the median initial HCG levels in CHMCF were significantly higher than in singleton molar pregnancy, the risk of GTN is similar, 25% versus 17%, respectively ($P = 0.63$). However, Suksai et al. [12] found 37% incidence of GTN after CHMCF in their study. The chances of developing GTN was higher in the group of females who had live birth as compared to those having poor perinatal outcomes [50.48 versus 23.08%, respectively ($P < 0.001$)]. Development of GTN was found in 15.8% (3/19) of females who had elective termination at the first trimester of pregnancy while it was 20.7% (12/58) in females who were in the second trimester of pregnancy. Since there is no statistically significant difference between early termination of pregnancy or continuation of pregnancy, so risk of post-molar GTN should not be an indication of terminating these pregnancies [12, 13]. Follow-up and chemotherapy will be same as follow-up of post-molar GTN following complete mole. Most of these patients require monotherapy as shown in a study by Sebire et al. [6]. In this study, 73% (11/15) of patients needed monochemotherapy while combination chemotherapy was given to four patients.

Patients with complete hydatidiform mole with live coexisting foetus can be given the option of continuation of pregnancy keeping in mind about strict foetomaternal surveillance. Even postpartum follow-up for post-molar GTN is very important for them and for which they should be adequately counselled and appropriately managed.

References

1. Bovicelli L, Ghi T, Pilu G, et al. Prenatal diagnosis of a complete mole coexisting with a dichorionic twin pregnancy: case report. Hum Reprod. 2004;19:1231–4.
2. Lai CY, Chan KY, Khoo US, et al. Analysis of gestational trophoblastic disease by genotyping and chromosome in situ hybridization. Mod Pathol. 2004;17:40–8.
3. Rohilla M, Singh P, Kaur J, et al. Individualistic approach to the management of complete hydatidiform mole with coexisting live fetus. Eur J Obstet Gynecol Reprod Biol. 2015;191:39–42.
4. Massardier J, Golfier F, Journet D, et al. Twin pregnancy with complete hydatidiform mole and coexistent fetus: obstetrical and oncological outcomes in a series of 14 cases. Eur J Obstet Gynecol Reprod Biol. 2009;143:84–7.
5. Wee L, Jauniaux E. Prenatal diagnosis and management of twin pregnancies complicated by a co-existing molar pregnancy. Prenat Diagn. 2005;25:772–6.
6. Sebire NJ, Foskett M, Paradinas FJ, et al. Outcome of twin pregnancies with complete hydatidiform mole and healthy co-twin. Lancet. 2002;359:2165–6.
7. Matsui H, Iitsuka Y, Ishii J, et al. Androgenetic complete mole coexistent with a live fetus. Gynecol Oncol. 1999;74:217–21.
8. Matsui H, Sekiya S, Hando T, et al. Hydatidiform mole coexistent with a twin live fetus: a national collaborative study in Japan. Hum Reprod. 2000;15:608–11.
9. Marcorelles P, Audrezet MP, Le Bris MJ, et al. Diagnosis and outcome of complete hydatidiform mole coexisting with a live twin fetus. Eur J Obstet Gynecol Reprod Biol. 2005;118:21–7.
10. Kihara M, Usui H, Tanaka H, Inoue H, Matsui H, Shozu M. Complicating preeclampsia as a predictor of poor survival of the fetus in complete hydatidiform mole coexistent with twin fetus. J Reprod Med. 2012;57:325–8.
11. Niemann I, Sunde L, Petersen LK. Evaluation of the risk of persistent trophoblastic disease after twin pregnancy with diploid hydatidiform mole and coexisting normal fetus. Am J Obstet Gynecol. 2007;197(45):e1–5.
12. Suksai et al. Complete hydatidiform mole with co-existing fetus: Predictors of live birth. Eur J Obstet Gynecol Reprod Biol. 2017;212:1–8.
13. Vaisbuch E, Ben-Arie A, Dgani R, et al. Twin pregnancy consisting of a complete hydatidiform mole and co-existent fetus: report of two cases and review of literature. Gynecol Oncol. 2005;98:19–23.

Management of Low-Risk Gestational Trophoblastic Neoplasia

8

Nomonde Mbatani

Gestational Trophoblastic Disease (GTD) is a rare disease. Worldwide, the incidences vary by regions with low rates found in some parts of South America, Europe, and North America [1] whilst countries in East-Asia report higher rates. Advances in prenatal imaging, immune-histological staining, and DNA ploidy technology help improve making a diagnosis [2–5].

GTN is the malignant form of GTD, encompasses (a) Invasive mole, (b) Choriocarcinoma, (c) PSTT, and (d) ETT.

8.1 GTD Risk Factors

- Extremes of maternal age [6, 7].
- Race: Indo-Asian race has been shown to have higher incidence and even in reports of Asian people residing in countries outside Asia the incidence is higher. A race may also be a proxy for persistent disease. Both the Asian race and extremes of age are closely associated with a complete molar pregnancy, in whom about 15% of patients develop gestational trophoblastic neoplasia (GTN) [8, 9].
- A history of a previous molar pregnancy also adds to the risk [1, 10].

The characteristic cytogenetic changes occur on the chorion, featuring as an abnormal proliferation of the trophoblast (either cytotrophoblast, syncytiotrophoblast, or intermediate trophoblast). The chorionic villi may undergo hydropic dilatation.

N. Mbatani (✉)
Groote Schuur Hospital, University of Cape Town, Cape Town, South Africa
e-mail: nomonde.mbatani@uct.ac.za

B. Nayak, U. Singh (eds.), *Gestational Trophoblastic Disease*,
https://doi.org/10.1007/978-981-33-4878-3_8

8.2 Gestational Trophoblastic Neoplasia

Gestational trophoblastic neoplasia (GTN) occurs as a complication of a prior molar pregnancy, a term pregnancy, or a miscarriage. Though GTN has varying potential from local invasion to distant metastasis, it is extremely chemosensitive and with high cure rate (90–100%).

Gestational trophoblastic neoplasia, also otherwise called persistent post-molar trophoblastic disease arises as the tumour cells continue to proliferate and produce βhCG, despite complete evacuation of the uterus. The FIGO diagnosis of post-molar GTN is made when three βhCG values increase by at least 10% over 2 weeks or plateaus (four readings that are within 10% range over 3 weeks and histological diagnosis of Choriocarcinoma [11]. In addition to the above recommended diagnostic criteria, the Charing Cross Hospital, incorporates an hCG level that is ≥20,000 IU/L 4 weeks after uterine evacuation. Similarly few centres do initiate chemotherapy when hCG remains positive 6 months post evacuation. However , the criteria of a positive value 6 months post evacuation has been removed from the FIGO list. A Brazilian retrospective survey of patients with CHM who were later started on single agent chemotherapy for GTN could not find any difference in outcomes or any increase in treatment failure between patients who had hCG levels below 20,000 IU/L at 4 weeks, compared to those with levels higher than 20,000 IU/L at the same time [12]. Patients with molar pregnancies, who are followed up and monitored with βhCG levels, the following risk factors should alert the medical practitioner to possible persistent disease:

- Uterine size is much larger than the estimated gestational age.
- Corpus luteal cysts more than 6 cm in size.
- Extremes of maternal age.
- GTD associated comorbid diseases such as hyperthyroidism and pre-eclampsia.
- Complete mole histology.
- βHCG value more than 100,000 Iu/mL at diagnosis.
- H/O Previous molar pregnancy.

After evacuation, 2–6% of partial moles and about 13–24% of complete molar gestation will progress to gestational trophoblastic neoplasia and require chemotherapy [13–16].

In other instances, complete molar tissue may invade deeply into the myometrium, the vagina, or sometimes spread to the lungs. Histologically, invasive molar tissue contains villous material that infiltrates these structures. This is the diagnostic feature that differentiates the invasive mole from choriocarcinoma, which bears no chorionic villi (see Table 8.1). However, histological confirmation of metastases should be avoided, as fatal bleeding may occur with the procedure. It is suggested that any woman in her reproductive age who presents with metastatic disease or with bizarre clinical presentation, the serum βhCG should be checked to exclude

Table 8.1 WHO risk scoring chart

Prognostic factor	0	1	2	4
Age	Younger than 40 years	40 years or older	–	–
Previous pregnancy	Hydatidiform mole	Abortion	Full term	–
Months since last pregnancy	Less than 4	4–6	7–12	More than 12
Pretreatment βHCG (IU/mL)	Less than 10^3	10^3 to 10^4	>10^4 to 10^5	>10^5
Largest tumour size, including uterus	Less than 3 cm	3 to <5 cm	5 cm or more	–
Site of metastasis	Lung	Spleen or kidney	Gastrointestinal tract	Brain, liver
Number of metastases	Zero	1–4	5–8	More than eight
Number of drugs used to treat the tumours that have not worked	None	None	One drug	Two or more drugs

GTN [17]. Moreover, intervals more than 4 months between the pregnancy and the GTN event are associated with undesirable outcomes [18].

Besides the FIGO anatomical staging, the WHO has a scoring system that predicts disease prognosis (see Table 8.1). Based on the score, GTN is classified as low risk and high risk. It is considered low risk if:

1. FIGO Stage 1 GTN (Disease confined to the uterus).
2. Stage 2 or 3 GTN with a WHO score of less than 7.

8.3 Pre-Treatment Evaluation

Once the diagnosis of GTN is established (following FIGO criteria), a metastatic work-up is done to stage and score the disease. In addition to routine haematological investigations that include the following CBC, LFT, and RFT. A chest X-ray is done to exclude lung metastasis. An ultrasound or a CT scan of the abdomen and pelvis (where available), to exclude pelvic extension of the disease, and to rule out liver and other abdominal organ metastasis. A CT chest is not mandatory if the chest X-ray (CXR) is normal, though micro-metastases in the range of ~40% of patients may be detected by CT scan. The presence of lung micro-metastasis does not influence the outcome [19]. When lung metastases are detected on CXR, a CT scan of the lungs and an MRI of the brain need to be done to exclude brain metastasis and widespread disease. However, for the purpose of risk scoring, only a chest X-ray may be used for counting the number of metastases [20].

8.4 Management of Low-Risk GTN

8.4.1 Chemotherapy in Low-Risk GTD

Single agent chemotherapy (either as MTX or Actinomycin-D) is used to treat low-risk disease. Methotrexate is an antifolate antimetabolite that inhibits DNA and RNA syntheses. Folinic acid replacement should be prescribed as rescue treatment when prescribing the drug. Used as first-line treatment in patients with low-risk disease, the response rates to Methotrexate may be as high as 72% [21]. Different Methotrexate dosage regimes have been proposed (see Table 8.1). Dactinomycin or Actinomycin D is an intravenous anti-neoplastic antibiotic. It acts by inhibiting RNA synthesis. Like Methotrexate, it can be used singly or as part of combination therapy in the treatment of GTN.

Although there is acceptance of the Dactinomycin and Methotrexate as first-line drugs, there is no consensus on the most effective dose for both drugs. The Gynecologic Oncology Group (GOG) carried out a phase 3 study comparing the two drugs [21]. Dactinomycin 1.25 mg/m^2, administered every 2 weeks seemed to achieve better complete response rates (CR) than Methotrexate. Contrary to the recommended 30–50 mg/m^2 Methotrexate dosing practice, all patients in the Methotrexate arm were offered a fixed dose of 30 mg/m^2, as earlier studies by the same group found no benefit in higher doses. Both drugs performed less well when the WHO scores were between 5 and 6 and when the diagnosis was choriocarcinoma. A recent Cochrane review endorses pulsed Dactinomycin as a better choice for low-risk disease [22]. Most south east Asian countries use the 8 day methotrexate folinic acid regimen because the regimen is safe with good response rates. Etoposide is widely used as the first choice for monotherapy in China. For patients with an intermediate WHO score of 5–6 and with Choriocarcinoma, there is 35% chance of cure with Methotrexate regimen. Multi-agent chemotherapy should be considered early, should resistance to single agent treatment be suspected [11, 23, 27]. This group should be carefully managed and change over to multidrug regimen should not be delayed as there is a risk of chemoresitance and loss of unnecessary drug cycles.

For patients who still remain hCG positive at 6 months, chemotherapy may be deferred as long as a drop in HCG is demonstrated [23]. FIGO cancer report 2018 has withdrawn this issue from the diagnostic criteria of GTN.

Regardless of treatment protocol followed, at least two more insurance courses of chemotherapy should be administered after normalisation of hCG [24].

Should the hCG value either plateau or rise during MTX regimen therapy reflecting resistance, it is better to switch to Actinomycin-D or combination chemotherapy depending on the level of hCG < 300 IU/L or > 300 IU/L, respectively [25].

The Risk of relapse is less than 5% after 1 year of successful treatment and often negligible beyond 1 year of remission [26].

8.4.2 Second-Line Treatment for Low-Risk GTN

Dactinomycin used singly is an effective option after failure of Methotrexate and would circumvent the side effects of multiple agent drug treatment [27, 28]. Golfier et al. in their review of 877 patients who were put on Dactinomycin due to failed Methotrexate use, observed that there is a group of patients who may despite low FIGO scores, still have a high likelihood to develop resistance to second-line Dactinomycin monotherapy [29]. These are patients who have had either a non-molar antecedent pregnancy or a histological diagnosis of a prior hydatid molar pregnancy, and a re-course becomes inevitable.

Follow-up—After completion of treatment monthly βhCG to be done for 12 months as remission after that is very low. Contraceptives are advised to prevent pregnancy during follow-up [29].

8.5 Surgery

A hysterectomy is seldom indicated as first-line treatment in patients with low-risk scores, unless there are no more fertility desires and the disease is confined to the uterus. The most common indication for a Hysterectomy is an uncontrollable uterine bleed [30], or chemo-resistant cases. A hysterectomy may be beneficial to women with advanced maternal age, especially when the hCG is markedly elevated as the risk of GTN is more than 50% [31]. A hysterectomy does not preclude routine post-treatment GTD follow-up. The role of second curettage in low-risk GTN in obviating chemotherapy is controversial. Role of second curettage has to be sought thoughtfully when the residual disease is confined to the endometrial cavity without any myometrial extension. Evidences are both in favour and against the procedure mostly in the score group of ≤ 4 [32, 33].

8.5.1 Pregnancy After Treatment of a Molar Pregnancy

Women who elect to become pregnant should be informed about a 10–20 fold risk of subsequent molar gestation after the management of molar pregnancy [7, 34, 35]. Women should be counselled to book early for antenatal care and have ultrasound imaging to exclude a possible repeat molar pregnancy, especially those who have been treated for a complete mole [15, 36]. Though follow-up is at least for 12 months, pregnancy may be allowed after 6 months in such patients. If pregnancy occurs during follow-up, termination is not advised. The placenta or products of conception should be sent for histopathological review. Serum hCG level should be obtained at 6 weeks after the completion of pregnancy to exclude occult trophoblastic disease.

8.6 Conclusion

Gestational Trophoblastic Diseases are rare. The diagnosis is in some instances difficult to reach and can be frustrating to affected individuals. Early diagnosis and follow-up are crucial. The prognosis following treatment is excellent. The chance of a normal full-term pregnancy after diagnosis is almost the same as in women, without a prior diagnosis of GTD [37].

FIGO Staging of Gestational trophoblastic Neoplasia

- Stage I—Disease confined to the uterus.
- Stage II—Disease outside the uterus but still confined to the pelvis.
- Stage III—Lung metastasis.
- Stage IV—Distant metastasis other than lungs.

Common low-risk disease drug regimens [35]

Methotrexate (MTX)

- **Weekly dose**: 30–50 mg/m^{2}intramuscularly
- **Two weekly doses**:

1. MTX 0.4 mg/kg [maximum 25 mg] daily for 5 days. Repeat after 2 weeks.

   OR

2. MTX 300 mg/m^2 intravenously every two weeks.

   OR

3. MTX—1 mg/kg on days 1, 3, 5, and 7 alternating with Folinic acid 15 mg PO/IM –0.1 mg/kg on days 2, 4, 6, 8. To be repeated 2 weekly [8 day regime].

Dactinomycin/actinomycin D:

1. 1.25 mg/m^{2}intravenously every 2 weeks
2. 0.5 mg daily × 5 days. Repeat every 2 weeks

Various single dose regimen in low-risk GTN-ESGO GTN-2018

8-day methotrexate/folinic acid	Methotrexate (1.0–1.5 mg/kg) intramuscular on days 1, 3, 5, 7 with folinic acid rescue 5 mg given 24 or 30 h later on (days 2, 4, 6, 8) repeated every 14 days.
5-day methotrexate	Methotrexate intravenous 0.4 mg/kg on days 1 to 5 (maximum, 25 mg/day) repeated every 14 days
Weekly methotrexate	**Methotrexate (50 mg/m^2) intramuscular repeated weekly**
5-day dactinomycin	Dactinomycin (10–12 mg/kg or 0.5 mg total dose) intravenous daily for 5 days repeated every 14 days
Pulsed dactinomycin	**BIweekly dactinomycin (a single 1.25 mg/m^2 IV dose every 2 weeks)**

References

1. Altieri A, Franceschi S, Ferlay J, Smith J, La Vecchia C. Epidemiology and aetiology of gestational trophoblastic diseases. Lancet Oncol. 2003;4:670–8.
2. Osterheld MC, Caron L, Meagher CP, Villemure K. Combination of immunohistochemistry and ploidy analysis to assist histopathological diagnosis of molar. Clin Med Pathol. 2008;1:61–7. https://doi.org/10.4137/cpath.s601.
3. Ronnett BM. Hydatidiform moles. Ancillary techniques to refine diagnosis. Arch Pathol Lab Med. 2018;142:1485–502. https://doi.org/10.5858/arpa.2018-0226-RA.
4. Hemming JD, Quirke P, Womack C, Wells M, Elston CW. Diagnosis of molar pregnancy and persistent trophoblastic disease by flow cytometry. J Clin Pathol. 1987;40:615–20.
5. Khashaba M, Arafa M, Elsalkh E, Hemida R, Kandil W. Morphological features and immunohistochemical expression of p57Kip2 in early molar pregnancies and their relations to the progression to persistent trophoblastic disease. J Pathol Transl Med. 2017;51(4):381–7. https://doi.org/10.4132/jptm.2017.04.28.
6. Gockley AA, Melamed A, Joseph NT, Clapp M, Berkowitz RS. Effect of race/ethnicity on risk of complete and partial molar pregnancy. Gynecol Oncol. 2016;140(3):470–3. https://doi.org/10.1016/j.ygyno.2016.01.005.
7. Bracken MB. Incidence and aetiology of hydatidiform mole: an epidemiological review. BJOG Int J Obstet Gynaecol. 1987;94:1123–35. https://doi.org/10.1111/j.1471-0528.1987.tb02311.x.
8. Lurain JR. Gestational trophoblastic disease I: epidemiology, pathology, clinical presentation and diagnosis of gestational trophoblastic disease, and management of hydatidiform mole. Am J Obstet Gynecol. 2010;203(6):531–9. https://doi.org/10.1016/j.ajog.2010.06.073.
9. Maestá I, Berkowitz RS, Goldstein DP, Bernstein MR, Ramírez LA, Horowitz NS. Relationship between race and clinical characteristics, extent of disease, and response to chemotherapy in patients with low-risk gestational trophoblastic neoplasia. Gynecol Oncol. 2015;138(1):50–4.
10. Feltmate CM, Grwdon WB, Wolfberg AJ, Goldstein DP, Genest DR, Chinchila ME, Berkowitz RS. Clinical characteristics of persistent gestational trophoblastic neoplasia after partial hydatidiform molar pregnancy. J Reprod Med. 2006;51(11):902–6.
11. Ngan HYS, Seckl MJ, Berkowitz RS, Xiang Y, Golfier F, Sekharan PK, et al. Update on the diagnosis and management of gestational trophoblastic disease. Int J Gynecol Obstet. 2018;143:79–85. https://doi.org/10.1002/ijgo.12615.
12. Braga A, Biscaro A, do Amaral Giordani JM, Viggiano M, Elias KM, Berkowitz RS, Seckl MJ. Does a human chorionic gonadotropin level of over 20,000 IU/L four weeks after uterine evacuation for complete hydatidiform mole constitute an indication for chemotherapy for gestational trophoblastic neoplasia? Eur J Obstet Gynecol Reprod Biol. 2018;223:50–5. https://doi.org/10.1016/j.ejogrb.2018.02.001.
13. Wiesma S, Kerkmeijer L, Bekkers R, Pyman J, Tan J, Quinn M. Persistent trophoblast disease following partial molar pregnancy. Aust New Zealand J Obstet Gynaecol. 2006;46(2):119–23. https://doi.org/10.1111/j.1479-828X.2006.00539.x.
14. Soares RR, Maesta I, Colon J. Complete molar pregnancy in adolescents from North and South America: clinical presentation and risk of gestational trophoblastic neoplasia. Gynecol Oncol. 2016;142:496–500.
15. Savage PM, Sita-Lumsden A, Dickson S, Iyer R, Everard J, Coleman R, et al. The relationship of maternal age to molar pregnancy incidence, risks for chemotherapy and subsequent pregnancy outcome. J Obstet Gynaecol. 2013;33(4):406–11. https://doi.org/10.3109/01443615.2013.771159.
16. Rice LW, Berkowitz RS, Lage J, et al. Persistent gestational trophoblastic tumor after partial hydatidiform mole. Gynecol Oncol. 1990;36(3):358–62. https://doi.org/10.1016/0090-8258(90)90142-8.
17. FIGO Oncology Committee. FIGO staging for gestational trophoblastic neoplasia 2000. FIGO oncology committee. Int J Gynaecol Obstet. 2002;77(3):285–7.

18. Ghaemmaghami F, Zarchi MK. Early onset of metastatic gestational trophoblastic disease after full-term pregnancy. Int J Biomed Sci. 2008;4(1):74–7.
19. Darby S, Jolley I, Pennington S, Hancock BW. Does chest CT matter in the staging of GTN? Gynecol Oncol. 2009;112:155–60.
20. Ngan HYS, Benedet JL, Bender HG, et al. FIGO staging for gestational trophoblastic neoplasia. Int J Gynaecol Obstet. 2002;77:285–7.
21. Khan F, Everard J, Ahmed S, Coleman RE, Aitken M, Hancock BW. Low-risk persistent gestational trophoblastic disease treated with low-dose methotrexate: efficacy, acute and long-term effects. Br J Cancer. 2003;89(12):2197–201. https://doi.org/10.1038/sj.bjc.6601422.
22. Alazzam M, Tidy J, Osborne R, Coleman R, Hancock BW, Lawrie TA. Chemotherapy for resistant or recurrent gestational trophoblastic neoplasia. Cochrane Database Syst Rev. 2016;1 https://doi.org/10.1002/14651858.CD008891.pub3.
23. Sita-Lumsden A, Short D, Lindsay I, Sebire NJ, Adjogatse D, Seckl MJ, Savage PM. Treatment outcomes for 618 women with gestational trophoblastic tumours following a molar pregnancy at the Charing Cross Hospital, 2000-2009. Br J Cancer. 2012;107:1810–4.
24. Braga A, Torres B, Burlá M, Maestá I, Sun S, et al. Is chemotherapy necessary for patients with molar pregnancy and human chorionic gonadotropin serum levels raised but falling at 6 months after uterine evacuation? Gynecol Oncol. 2016;143(3):558–64. https://doi.org/10.1016/j.ygyno.2016.09.012.
25. Taylor F, Short D, Winter MC, TIDY J, Savage PM, Sarwar N, et al. A retrospective study to evaluate single agent methotrexate treatment in low risk gestational choriocarcinoma in the United Kingdom. Gynecol Oncol. 2015;136(2):258–63.
26. Lybol C, Sweep FCGJ, Harvey R, Mitchell H, Short D, Thomas CMG, et al. Relapse rates after two versus three consolidation courses of methotrexate in the treatment of low-risk gestational trophoblastic neoplasia. Gynecol Oncol. 2012;125(3):576–9.
27. Prouvot C, Golfier F, Massadier J, You B, Lotz JP, Patrier S, et al. Efficacy and safety of second-line 5-day dactinomycin in case of methotrexate failure for gestational trophoblastic neoplasia. Int J Gynecol Cancer. 2018;28(5):1038–44. https://doi.org/10.1097/IGC.0000000000001248.
28. McNeish IA, Strickland S, Holden L, Rustin GJS, Foskett M, Seckl MJ, Newlands ES. Low-risk persistent gestational trophoblastic disease: outcome after initial treatment with low-dose methotrexate and folinic acid from 1992 to 2000. J Clin Oncol. 2002;20(7):1838–44. https://doi.org/10.1200/JCO.2002.07.166.
29. Golfier F, Goffin F, Massardier J, Bolze P. Treatment of gestational throphoblastic neoplasia. ESGO gynaecological oncology textbook, 3rd ed.; 2016. https:www.esgo.org/media/2016/12/ESGO-3rd-edition-list-of-authors.
30. Eoh KJ, Chung YS, Yim GW, Nam EJ, Kim S, Kim SW, Kim YT. Role of surgical therapy in the management of gestational trophoblastic neoplasia. Obstetr Gynecol Sci. 2015;58(4):277. https://doi.org/10.5468/ogs.2015.58.4.277.
31. Elias KM, Shoni M, Bernstein M, Golstein DP, Berkowitz RS. Complete hydatidiform mole in women aged 40 to 49 years. J Reprod Med. 2012;57(5–6):254–8.
32. Osborne RJ, Filiac VL, Schink JC, Mannel RS, Behbakhi K, et al. Second curettage for low-risk nonmetastatic gestational trophoblastic neoplasia. Obstet Gynecol. 2016;128(3):535–42. 2
33. Reda H, Elvira LV, Basem EL-D, Mahammad A, Eman T, et al. Second uterine curettage and number of chemotherapy courses in post molar gestational trophoblastic neoplasia. Obstet Gynecol. 2019;133(5):1024–31.
34. New zealand Gynecologic Cancer group guidelines. 15/01/2014 Gestational throphoblastic Disease. https://nationalwomenshealth.adhb.govt.nz/assets/uploads/Gestational-Throphoblastic-Disease-Guidelines.pdf.
35. Sebire NJ, Fisher RA, Foskett M, Rees H, Seckl MJ, Newlands ES. Risk of recurrent hydatidiform mole and subsequent pregnancy outcome following complete or partial hydatidiform molar pregnancy. BJOG. 2003;110(1):22–6. PMID: 12504931.
36. Lorigan PC, Sharma S, Bright N, Coleman RE, Hancock BW. Characteristics of women with recurrent molar pregnancies. Gynecol Oncol. 2000;78(3):288–92.
37. Garrett LA, Garner E, Feltmate CM, Goldstein DP, Berkowitz RS. Subsequent pregnancy outcomes in patients with molar pregnancy and persistent gestational trophoblastic neoplasia. Obstet Gynecol Surv. 2008;11:704–5. https://doi.org/10.1097/01.ogx.0000335639.50781.

High-Risk Gestational Trophoblastic Neoplasia

9

K. Kalaichelvi

9.1 Introduction

Gestational trophoblastic disease (GTD) comprises a spectrum of diseases which includes benign and malignant neoplasms arising from villous and extravillous trophoblasts. Gestational trophoblastic neoplasia (GTN) denotes malignant complications of trophoblasts which include Invasive mole, Choriocarcinoma (CC), Placental Site Trophoblastic Tumor (PSTT), and Epithelioid Trophoblastic Tumor (ETT).

GTN is unique because it is the only disease that can be cured by chemotherapy alone and also does not require histopathological proof for treatment. The tumor marker beta-human chorionic gonadotrophin (hCG) is 100% sensitive in diagnosis, treatment monitoring, and follow-up of GTN. GTN is diagnosed usually during follow-up of a molar pregnancy. Fifty percent of GTN follow molar pregnancy, 20% can occur after a spontaneous abortion, 5% after ectopic pregnancy, and 25% following term pregnancy. Metastatic GTN occurs in 4% of patients after complete molar pregnancy.

PSTT and ETT however develop after term deliveries or non-molar abortions in 95% of the cases [1, 2].

The GTN is classified as Low-risk and High-risk GTN according to FIGO 2002 staging system. When the score is ≤6, it is low-risk GTN and ≥ 7 are grouped as High-risk GTN (Stage IV and Stage II and III with a score of ≥7). Ultrahigh-risk GTN is defined when the score is >12 [3, 4]. The management of High-risk GTN is by combination chemotherapy. The cure rate is 80–90% as it is highly sensitive to chemotherapy. However, 10–20% of women with high-risk GTN die subsequently due to drug-resistant disease [2].

K. Kalaichelvi (✉)
Department of Medical Oncology, Madras Medical College, Chennai, Tamil Nadu, India

B. Nayak, U. Singh (eds.), *Gestational Trophoblastic Disease*,
https://doi.org/10.1007/978-981-33-4878-3_9

Table 9.1 FIGO anatomic staging for gestational trophoblastic neoplasia [3, 4]

Stage I	Disease confined to the uterus
Stage II	GTN extends outside of the uterus but is limited to the genital structures (adnexa, vagina, broad ligament)
Stage III	GTN extends to the lungs, with or without known genital tract
Stage IV	All other metastatic sites

Note: FIGO, International Federation of Gynaecology and Obstetrics; GTN, Gestational trophoblastic neoplasia

Table 9.2 Modified WHO prognostic scoring system as adapted by FIGO [3, 4]

Scores	0	1	2	4
Age	<40	>40	–	–
Antecedent pregnancy	Mole	Abortion	Term	–
Interval months from index pregnancy	<4	4–7	7–13	>13
Pretreatment serum hCG (IU/L)	<1000	<10,000	<100,000	>100,000
Largest tumor size (including uterus)	–	3 to <5 cm	>5 cm	–
Site of metastases	Lung	Spleen/kidney	GI	Liver/brain
Number of metastases	–	1–4	5–8	>8
Previous failed chemotherapy	–	–	Single drug	Two or more drugs

FIGO, International Federation of Gynaecology and Obstetrics; WHO, World Health Organization

The FIGO staging/modified WHO scoring system is most commonly used for classifying patients with GTN and this revised FIGO staging was published in 2002 which recommended the use of a universal GTN risk stratification [3, 4]. FIGO 2002 has an anatomical staging system and a modified WHO scoring system (Tables 9.1 and 9.2). The staging should be reported in Roman numeral followed by the score in Arabic numerals separated by a colon, e.g., stage II: 3, stage IV: 8.

This stage and score will be allotted for each patient. PSTT and ETT are not scored but anatomic staging can be given as these entities differ in their behavior from regular post-molar GTN.

9.2 Typical Presenting Symptoms and Clinical Features

Though presenting features of GTN are typical to the severity of the disease, sometimes patients may present with very minimal or no symptoms in spite of the presence of widespread disease. This should be kept in mind while dealing with a patient with GTN as early diagnosis and prompt appropriate treatment is curable in most instances.

- History and physical exam
- Serum BHCG
- CBC,RFT,LFT,sugar,viral markers
- USG with Doppler-invasion into myometrium,vascularity, PI and RI, Theca Lutein cysts, Liver mets
- Chest xray
- If chest xray is negative, CT Scan chest
- If Lung mets are noted CT Abdomen and MRI Brain

Extensive lung metastasis can present with cough, dyspnea, and hemoptysis. Minimal or few lung metastases do not produce any symptoms. Pleural effusion, usually hemorrhagic, can present with dyspnea.

Some patients may present with symptoms of raised intracranial pressure like convulsions, headache, dizziness, and hemiplegia due to brain metastasis.

PSTT and ETT may present with irregular bleeding or amenorrhea following an antecedent term pregnancy. Serosanguinous or whitish particulate discharge can occur in patients with epithelioid trophoblastic tumor. There are reported cases of nephrotic syndrome and virilizing syndrome associated with these conditions.

Clinical exam may show an enlarged uterus, which may be irregular with or without bleeding. Sometimes a vaginal nodule can be made out; hence, pelvic examination should be done gently to avoid bleeding. Large theca lutein cysts can be palpated in the lower abdomen. Signs of raised intracranial pressure should be noted in patients with a history of headache and vomiting.

9.3 Diagnosis and Investigations Before Chemotherapy

Initial detailed history regarding the antecedent pregnancy and physical exam should be done with special precaution during a pelvic exam. The presence of a vaginal nodule should be looked for as it can start bleeding even with a rough vaginal exam. Serum hCG assay in standardized lab should be done along with routine investigations like renal, hepatic function tests, complete blood count, serum uric acid, electrolytes, sugar and viral markers like HBsAG, HCV, HIV. A chest X-ray to look for lung metastasis can be done, and if there is no metastasis, a CT scan chest can be done in high-risk GTN. If there are lung metastasis in the CT chest, CT of the abdomen and an MRI of the brain should be done to rule out liver, GIT, and brain metastasis as 20% of patients with lung metastasis can also have brain metastasis. An Ultrasonography (USG) of the pelvis combined with a Doppler study is helpful in evaluating the extent of uterine involvement and also invasion into the myometrium. Presence of low PI and RI (pulsatility and Resistive index) <1 is indicative of low resistance circulation characteristic of persistent trophoblastic disease and indicative of methotrexate resistance. USG also detects the presence of theca-lutein cysts and liver metastasis.

Repeat dilatation and curettage is contraindicated as it increases the risk of perforation, hemorrhage, and dissemination.

CSF hCG analysis is rarely necessary as high-resolution MRI of the brain is sufficient to identify CNS metastasis. PET-CT scan is not recommended as first-line investigations and it does not alter the management but may be useful to accurately identify metabolically active drug-resistant disease or viable metastasis and to help decide tumor resectability.

9.3.1 Treatment

Patients with high-risk GTN should receive combination chemotherapy. Historically, the combination chemotherapy given was MAC regimen (Methotrexate, Actinomycin D and cyclophosphamide or chlorambucil), and reported cure rates were between 63 and 71% [5–7]. Later CHAMOCA (cyclophosphamide, Hydroxyurea, Actinomycin D, methotrexate with folinic acid, vincristine, and doxorubicin) regimen was used with a remission rate of 80% [8]. However, in a randomized trial comparing MAC and CHAMOCA regimens in high-risk cases, it was found that the MAC regimen produced more cure rates (95%) than CHAMOCA (70%) and the MAC regimen was less toxic [9]. In 1980, when Etoposide was found to be effective in GTN, the EMA-CO regimen (Table 9.3) was designed by Newlands et al. and reported 80% complete clinical response in patients with high-risk GTN as primary chemotherapy and 82% survival with minimal toxicity in 72 patients [10]. Since then several studies have reported complete remission and survival rates over 80% with the EMA-CO regimen.

A Korean study compared MAC, CHAMOCA, and EMA-CO and showed remission rates of 67.5, 76.2, and 90.6%, respectively, proving that EMA-CO is the effective chemotherapy in high-risk GTN [11].

Long-term results of EMA-CO have shown an overall survival of 93% when this regimen was used as primary therapy [12]. The high response rates and good long-term survival rates and minimal acute and long-term side effects makes EMA-CO as the primary regimen of choice for high-risk GTN patients. There are reports on using the EMA part of EMA-CO omitting cyclophosphamide and vincristine resulting in complete remissions ranging from 71 to 78% [13].

EMA-CO is administered on alternate weeks and repeated once in 14 days. The dose intensity of the schedule should be maintained to prevent the development of drug resistance. Once remission is achieved, 2–4 cycles should be given

Table 9.3 EMA-CO regimen [11]

EMA-C0	Etoposide	100 mg/m^2	D1 & D2
	ActD	350 mcg/ m^2	D1 & D2
	MTX	100 mg/m^2 iv bolus, 200 mg/m^2–12 h infusion	D1
	Folinic acid	15 mg PO q12 h × 4 doses (24 h from MTX bolus)	D2
	Cyclophosphamide	600 mg/m^2	D8
	Vincristine	1 mg/m^2	D8

after the first normal hCG to prevent a relapse. If properly given, the EMA-CO regimen is well tolerated, the need for growth factor is very limited. The incidence of mucositis is <10%. Serum hCG should be measured before each cycle of EMA-CO and if there is plateauing of hCG values, a change of regimen is required. Serum hCG should come to normal by the fourth cycle. If it remains elevated even after four cycles, it is unlikely that they will achieve complete remission. In a study using the hCG regression curve, they found that an hCG value of ≥118.6 mIU/ml before the fifth cycle was highly predictive of EMA-CO resistance [14]. Patients with a long duration of disease (>12 months), more than two or three metastatic sites (brain, liver, GI tract) and ineffective prior chemotherapy were predictive for developing resistance or failure of EMA-CO regimen. In patients with high-risk GTN with high tumor volume and poor performance status, induction with EP (Etoposide100 mg/m^2 and cisplatin 20 mg/m^2) one or two weekly courses can be given before starting EMA-CO which reduces early mortality. Most probably she belongs to ultrahigh-risk GTN, which is dealt with separately in another chapter.

Salvage Regimens for High Risk GTN

1. EMA-EP
2. TP/TE
3. BEP
4. PVB
5. VIP
6. APE
7. FA
8. FAEV
9. ICE

Immunotherapy with Pembrolizumab

Those who fail the EMA-CO regimen should be treated with other salvage regimens. About 20% of high-risk patients will progress on or after primary chemotherapy. The salvage rate depends on effective chemotherapy and it is around 88% in a study [15]. The salvage regimens (Table 9.4) which are widely used are EMA-EP (Etoposide, Methotrexate, ActimoycinD, alternating with Etoposide and Cisplatin), TP/TE (Paclitaxel, Cisplatin alternating with Paclitaxel and Etoposide), BEP (Bleomycin, Etoposide Cisplatin) 5), ICE (Ifosfamide, Carboplatin, and Etoposide), VIP (Vinblastin, Ifosfamide, Cisplatin), APE (Actinomycin D, Cispltain, Etoposide), FA (5 Flurouracil, Actinomycin D), and FAEV (5 Floxuridine, Actinomycin, Etoposide, Vincristine). The most commonly used salvage regimen is EMA-EP (Substituting Cyclophosphamide, vincristine with Cisplatin and Etoposide) giving a remission rate of 70–80% [16]. Renal and hematological toxicity should be managed carefully and the growth factor can be used to manage myelosuppression. The EP part can be given on days 1 and 2 followed by EMA on days 8 and 9 which is much easier to manage

Table 9.4 Salvage regimens [15]

Regimen	Drug	Dose	Day
EMA-EP (q 14 days)	Etoposide	100 mg/m^2	D1 & D2
	ActD	350 mcg/m^2	
	MTX	100 mg/m^2 iv bolus, 200 mg/m^2—12 h infusion	D1–D2
	Folinic acid	15 mg PO q12 h × 4 doses (24 h from MTX bolus)	D2
	Cisplatin	60 mg/m^2	D8
	Etoposide	100 mg/m^2	D8
TP/TE (q 15 days)	Paclitaxel	135 mg/m^2	D1
	Cisplatin	60 mg/m^2	D1
	Paclitaxel	135 mg/m^2	D15
	Etoposide	50 mg/m^2	D15
BEP (q 21 days)	Bleomycin	30 unit	D1
	Etoposide	100 mg/m^2	D1–D5
	Cisplatin	20 mg/m^2	D1–D5
PVB (q 21 days)	Cisplatin	100 mg/m^2	Divided dose for D1–D3
	Vinblastine	0.11 mg/kg/day	D1–D2
	Bleomycin	30 mg	D1
VIP (q 21 days)	Vinblastine	0.11 mg/mg/day	D1–D2
	Ifosfamide	1.4 g/m^2	D1–D3
	Cisplatin	100 mg/m^2	ddD1–D3

the toxicity (EP/EMA) [17]. The other salvage regimen (TP/TE regimen) results in survival rates of 70–75% with manageable toxicity and use of growth factor support [16, 18]. BEP regimen is also used in resistant GTN and remission rates around 74% are reported [19]. Other salvage regimens are PVB (vinblastine, cisplatin, and bleomycin), ICE (ifosfamide, carboplatin, etoposide), VIP (vinblastine, ifosfamide, cisplatin) can be used in second- or third-line setting. The FA and FAEV regimen are used mainly in China. The FAEV regimen produces a 60% remission rate as a salvage regimen [20]. The high-dose chemotherapy with autologous stem-cell transplant can be tried in resistant GTN cases after failure of salvage chemotherapy with success rates around 50% [21] The high-dose regimens used are ICE, EC (etoposide, cyclophosphamide), and EP (etoposide, cisplatin).

Recently immunotherapy with Pembrolizumab has been reported in chemoresistant GTN [22]. Successful treatment of three out of four drug-resistant GTN patients with Pembrolizumab by Michel J Seckl et al. at Charing Cross Hospital, London, makes immunotherapy a life-saving treatment. The efficacy and favorable toxicity profile of Pembrolizumab makes it an alternative to high-dose chemotherapy. However, the risk of permanent infertility due to lasting anti-trophoblast immunity is a concern. Tumor-infiltrating lymphocytes and HLA-G expression might identify responders.

9.3.2 Placental Site Trophoblastic Tumor (PSTT)/Epithelioid Trophoblastic Tumor (ETT)

Placental site trophoblastic tumor and Epithelioid Trophoblastic Tumor are forms of GTN, arising from intermediate trophoblast (PSTT arises from implantation site trophoblast and ETT arises from chorionic type trophoblast), constituting 1–2% of all GTN, which can occur after any type of gestation [23]. It produces less quantity of hCG and is less chemosensitive. Hence, surgery is the mainstay of treatment. They are associated with less vascular invasion, necrosis, and hemorrhage, and have a propensity for lymphatic metastasis. Most cases follow term pregnancy. They may present with abnormal vaginal bleeding with varying periods of amenorrhea, and metastasis to various organs. Rarely, they present with galactorrhea, virilization, nephrotic syndrome, Polycythemia, and cutaneous metastases. HCG levels are often low; they range between 100 and 1000 miu/l. Rarely higher titers are also reported. Poor prognostic factors are interval > 2 years from antecedent pregnancy, Mitotic count >5/10 HPF, extensive necrosis and extension outside the uterus. Hysterectomy is the choice. Combination chemotherapy can be given after surgery till hCG remission is achieved. Cure rates are 80–90% with proper management. Epithelioid trophoblastic tumor is a rare variant of PSTT and treatment is the same as that of PSTT.

9.3.3 Role of Surgery

For resistant GTN cases, surgical option should be considered.

Preoperative imaging studies such as Ultrasound, MRI, Arteriography, and Positron **Emission Tomography with CT fusion imaging (PET-CT Scan)** may be helpful in identifying the site of residual tumor and help in surgical planning.

If the resistant disease is present in the uterus, a hysterectomy may be performed to remove the focus of drug-resistant disease.

If the woman desires fertility, local uterine resection of the tumor can be attempted. The future risk of uterus rupture during pregnancy should be explained.

If the resistant focus is found in the lungs, thoracotomy and resection of metastases can be done. Tomada et al. proposed the following criteria to predict successful pulmonary resection: (1) Patient is a good surgical candidate; (2) Primary malignancy is controlled; (3) Pulmonary metastasis limited to one lung; (4) No evidence of other metastatic sites; and (5) HCG level is <1000 miu/ml [24]. The success rate is high if all five criteria are met and it is zero if four or less than four are present. Serum hCG should become undetectable within 2 weeks after pulmonary resection of metastasis.

9.3.4 Follow-up

High-risk GTN should be followed up with monthly hCG for 2 years after remission and annually thereafter. Recurrences are around 3–9% which occurs within the first

1 year after completion of treatment. Contraception for 2 years should be advised and an oral contraceptive pill is safe to use. Fertility is not impaired in young women and also there is no increased incidence of congenital malformations. Confirmation of pregnancy with USG and estimation of serum hCG 6 weeks after delivery should be done to make sure that there is no evidence of GTD [1].

9.3.5 Long-Term Toxicity of Chemotherapy

Women who receive combination chemotherapy for GTN are likely to develop early menopause. Menopause gets advanced by 3 years after combination chemotherapy and 1 year after single-agent therapy [25].

The risk of developing a second malignancy is also increased in GTN patients who receive combination chemotherapy with alkylating agents and etoposide. A study has reported a relative risk (RR) of 16.6 for developing Acute Myeloid Leukemia and 4.6 relative risk for colon cancer, 3.4 for melanoma, and 5.79 for breast cancer in women surviving more than 25 years. If combination chemotherapy is given for less than 6 months, there may not be a risk for second cancers [26].

9.3.6 Psychosocial Effects

Women with GTN may experience mood disturbances, marital and sexual problems, and anxiety regarding future pregnancy. The psychological trauma of going through treatment may last long even after the follow-up period. Counseling is required for all women to gain confidence about the curability of the condition and future fertility preservation.

References

1. Goldstein DP, Berkowitz RS. Current management of gestational trophoblastic neoplasia. Haematol Oncol Clin. 2012;26(1):30–1.
2. Ngan HY, Kohorn EI, Cole LA, Kurman RJ, Kim SJ, Lurain JR, et al. Trophoblastic disease. Int J Gynaecol Obstet. 2012;119(Suppl 2):S130–6.
3. Kohorn E1. The new FIGO 2000 at risk factors scoring system for gestational trophoblastic disease; description and critical amendment intro. J Gynaec Cancer. 2001;11:73–7.
4. Ngan HY, Bender H, Benedet JL, et al. Gestational trophoblastic neoplasma, FIGO 2000 staging and classification. Tmt J Gynaecol Obstet. 2003;83:175–7.
5. Berkowitz RS, Goldstein DP, Bernstein MR. Modified triple chemotherapy in the management of high risk metastatic gestational trophoblastic tumours. Gynaecol Oncol. 1984;19:173–81.
6. Gorden AN, Gershenson DM, Copeland LJ, et al. High risk metastatic gestational trophoblastic disease. Obstet Gynaecol. 1985;65:550–6.
7. Lurain JR, Brewer JI. Treatment of high risk gestational trophoblastic disease with methotraxate, actinomycin D and cyclophosphamide chemotherapy. Obstet Gynaecol. 1985;65:830–4.
8. Begent RHJ, Bagshawe KD. The management of high-risk choriocarcinoma. Semin Oncol. 1982;9:198–203.

9. Curry SL, Blessing JA, Disaia PJ, et al. A perspective randomized comparison of methotrexate, actinomycin D and chlorambucil (MAC) versus modified Bagshawe regimen in "poor prognosis" gestational trophoblastic disease. Obstet Gynaecol. 1989;73:357–62.
10. Newlands ES, Bagshawe KD, Begent RHJ, et al. Results with EMA/CO (etoposide, methotextrate, actinomycin D, cyclophosphamide, vincristine) regimen in high risk gestational trophoblastic tumours, 1979–1989. Br J Obstet Gynaecol. 1991;98:550–7.
11. Kim SJ, Bae SN, Kim JH, et al. Effects of multiagent chemotherapy at independent risk factors in the treatment of high risk GTT-25 years of experiences of KRI-TRD. Int J Gynaecol Obstet. 1998;60:S85–96.
12. Lurain JR, Singh DK, Schink JC. Management of metastatic high risk gestational trophoblastic neoplasia FIGO stages II-IV: risk factors score ≥7. J Reprod Med. 2010; 55:199–207.
13. Matsui H, Suzuka K, Iitsuka Y, et al. Combination chemotherapy with methotextrate, etoposide and actinomycin D for high risk gestational trophoblastic tumours. Gynaecol Oncol. 2000;78:28–31.
14. Rattanaturi A, Boonyapipat S, Supasinth Y. Human chronic gonadotropin (HCG) regression curve for predicting response to EMA/CO (etoposide, methotextrate, actinomycin D, cyclophosphamide and vincristine) regimen in gestational trophoblastic neoplasia. Asian Pac J Cancer Prev. 2015;16:5037–41.
15. Newlands ES. The management of recurrent and drug resistant gestational trophoblastic neoplasia (GTN). Best Prac Res Clin Obstet Gynaecol. 2003;17(6):905–23.
16. Wang J, Short D, Safire NJ, Lindsay I, Newlands ES, et al. Salvage chemotherapy of relapsed or high risk gestational trophoblastic neoplasia (GTN) with paclitaxel/cisplatin alternating with paclitaxel/etoposide (TP/TE). Ann Oncol. 2008;19:1578–83.
17. Han SN, Amant F, Leuinen K, et al. EP–EMA regimen (etoposide, cisplatin with etoposide, methotextrate al dectmonycn) in a series of 18 women with gestational trophoblastic neoplasia Int. J Gynaecol Cancer. 2012;22:875–80.
18. Ostorne R, Covens A, Mirchandani D, Gernlath A. Successful salvage of relapsed high risk gestational trophoblastic neoplasia patients using a novel paclitaxel containing doublet. J Reprod Med. 2004;49:655–61.
19. Lurain JR, Nejad B. Secondary chemotherapy for high risk gestational trophoblastic neoplasia. Gynaecol Oncol. 2005;97:618–23.
20. Feng F, Xiang Y, Wan X, Geng S, Wang T. Salvage combination schemotherapy with floxuridine, dactinomycin, etoposide, and vincristine (FAEV) for patients withrelapsed/chemoresistant gestational trophoblastic neoplasia. Ann Oncol. 2011;22:1588–94.
21. Yamamoto E, Niimi K, Fujikake K, Nishida T, Murata M, et al. High -dose chemotherapy with autologous peripheral stem cell transplantation for choriocarcinoma. A case report and literature review. Mol Clin Oncol. 2016;5:660–4.
22. Ghorani E, Kaur B, Fisher RA, Shest D, Joneborg U, Carlson JW, Akarca A, Marafioti T, Quezale SA, Sarwar N, Seckl MJ. Pembrolizumab is effective for drug-resistant gestational trophoblastic neoplasia. 2017;390:P2343–5. www.thelancet.com
23. Hyman DM, Bakio SL, Gualtiere G, Carr C, Grisham RN, Makker V, et al. Placental site trophoblastic tumour analysis of presentation, treatment and outcome. Gynaecol Oncol. 2013;129(1):58–62.
24. Tomada Y, Arii Y, Kaseki S, Asai Y, Gotoh S, et al. Surgical indications for resection in pulmonary metastasis of choriocarcinoma. Cancer. 1980;46:2723–50.
25. Seckl MJ, GJS R. Late toxicity after therapy for gestational trophoblastic tumors. In: Hancock BW, Newlands ES, Berkowitz RS, Cole LA, editors. Gestational trophoblastic disease. 3rd ed. London: International Society for the Study of Trophoblastic Disease; 2003. p. 470–84.
26. Rustin GJS, Newlands ES, Lutz JM, Holden Bagshawe KD, Hiscox JG, et al. Combination but not single agent chemotherapy for gestational trophoblastic tumours (GTT) increase the evidence of second tumours. I Clin Omol. 1996;14:2769–73.

Further Reading

Gestational trophoblastic disease 4th edition (2015) Edited by B. W. Hancock, M. J. Seckl and R. S. Berrowitz Robert (ISSTD Book- available free on ISSTD home page).

Schink JC, Lurain JR. Gestrational trophoblastic diceses molar breagency and gestrational neoplasia in Chapter 27. In: Principles and practice of gynecologic oncology, 6th ed.; 2013. p. 886–908.

M. J. Seckl, N. J. Sebire, R. A. Fisher, F. Golfier, L. Massuger, C. Sessa Gestational trophoblastic disease: ESMO Clinical Practice Guidelines for diagnosis, treatment and follow up, On behalf of ESMO Guidelines working group. Ann Oncol. 2013; 24 Suppl 6:vi39–50.

Ultrahigh-Risk Gestational Trophoblastic Neoplasia

10

S. K. Giri, Bhagyalaxmi Nayak, and K. Kalaichelvi

Gestational trophoblastic neoplasia (GTN) is divided into low-risk and high-risk categories depending on the score of 0 to ≤6 or ≥ 7, respectively, in the FIGO/WHO scoring system in terms of management strategies. As evidenced from the scoring table, the lowest is 0 and the highest score is 25. A score of 6 or less is low-risk disease and is treated by single-agent chemotherapy. A score of 7 or greater is high-risk disease and needs combination chemotherapy. The overall survival (OS) in low-risk rate is almost 100%, and about 80–90% in high-risk diseases [1] Risk score 5–6 and diagnosis of Choriocarcinoma are associated with increased risk of resistance to single-agent chemotherapy. These situations need reconsideration for multi-agent chemotherapy [2]. Ironically, the diagnosis of Choriocarcinoma, though does have worse prognosis, is not included in the scoring system. It is observed that patients with high scores ≥13 with multiple metastases including that of the brain, liver do have poor prognosis, more so if treated upfront with conventional multi-agent chemotherapy as commonly followed in high-risk patients [2, 3]. The poor result and early death after chemotherapy is attributed to fatal haemorrhage or organ failure due to tumour lysis from the high disease burden in the liver, brain, and lungs. To better understand and define these issues of poor survival and complications, these patients are grouped and managed under the heading of **"ultrahigh-risk GTN"** [2, 4].

S. K. Giri (✉)
PG Department of Gynaecologic Oncology, A.H. Post Graduate Institute of Cancer, Cuttack, India

B. Nayak
Associate Professor, Department of Gynaecologic Oncology, Regional Cancer Center, Cuttack, India

K. Kalaichelvi
Department of Medical Oncology, Madras Medical College, Chennai, Tamil Nadu, India

B. Nayak, U. Singh (eds.), *Gestational Trophoblastic Disease*,
https://doi.org/10.1007/978-981-33-4878-3_10

10.1 Features of Presumptive Diagnosis of Ultrahigh-Risk GTN [5]

Once all or some of the following features are present, it creates an alarm for the disease condition:

- Antecedent pregnancy interval of >2.8 years
- β-hCG >1,000,000 mIU/ml
- Profuse vaginal bleeding
- Multiple (>20) metastases in lungs with haemoptysis
- Extensive liver metastases
- Brain metastases
- Suspected/confirmed diagnosis of Choriocarcinoma

ULRA HIGH - RISK GTN: Score ≥13

- Pathological or suspected choriocarcinoma,
- Multiple (>20) lung mets or associated with hemoptytsis
- Brain metastasis
- Large volume liver metastases
- Profuse vaginal bleeding
- HCG >10,00,000 IU/L
- Interval from antecedent pregnancy >2.8.yrs

10.2 Management

When scoring shows ultrahigh-risk disease, urgent evaluation should be done to prevent early death, as the disease evolves very fast. In addition to clinical examination and routine investigations, she should have a baseline ultrasound with colour Doppler study of the pelvis, CT scan of chest; abdomen and pelvis, MRI of the brain should be urgently done to assess the extent of the disease. Biopsy of any suspected lesion should be avoided. Lumbar puncture may be done when the procedure proves to be safe from the result of the above investigations. The CSF thus obtained can be subjected to hCG, cytology, protein, and glucose. An hCG CSF:Serum ratio of more than 1:60 is suggestive of CNS involvement [5].

Once the evaluation is done, she should be transferred to the centres with experience and facility for ICU care. Chemotherapy by an experienced oncologist should be started as soon as possible. If standard chemotherapy like EMA-CO regimen is initiated in such a patient with a high tumour burden, she may experience severe bleeding from the site of metastasis with sudden collapse, metabolic acidosis, bone marrow depression, multiple organ failure and septicaemia. Any or all of these complications can lead to early death [2].

Low-dose induction chemotherapy like Etoposide 100 mg/m^2 and Cisplatin 20 mg/m^2 on days 1 and 2 should be started and repeated every week for 1–3 weeks [6]. Initiation of low-dose induction chemotherapy reduces the tumour volume gradually, so that significant bleeding from the organs with high-volume metastases is minimised. By that time the general condition of most patients improves, so that standard chemotherapy (EMA-CO) regimen can be initiated. After normalisation of hCG, consolidation therapy should continue for 3–4 cycles. This approach reduces early death from 7.8 to 0.7% in all high-risk cases [7]. The use of chemotherapy in such types of highly chemosensitive tumours can result in tumour lysis syndrome. This situation can be reduced by prompt hydration, maintaining electrolyte balance, and maintenance of renal function and initiation of allopurinol therapy [5].

In cases of metastatic disease **in the brain**, after induction therapy with EP, the Methotrexate dose in the EMA-CO regimen is increased to 1 gm/m^2 given over 24 h (EMA-CNS), so that the drug can cross the blood–brain barrier. Intrathecal methotrexate 12.5 mg can be an option with the doses of CO, depending upon the situation [8]. In such a situation, some centres do try whole-brain radiotherapy 15 fractions at the dose of 200cGY/fraction or stereotactic/gamma knife radiation in residual brain lesions, though there is no improved outcome [8, 9]. Whole-brain radiotherapy (WBRT) along with chemotherapy can be given but can result in long-term neurotoxicity in the form of reduction in intellectual capacity [10]. Surgery can be done for isolated lesions or to control bleeding from metastasis. Craniotomy may sometimes be required to release intracranial pressure.

Liver metastases are usually part of large-volume disease and very high hCG levels. These patients may have diseases involving other organs like the lung, vagina and brain. They may not have symptoms related to liver involvement at all. Bakri et al. noted that only 5 of 19 patients (26%) with liver metastasis presented with liver-related complaints such as jaundice, intraabdominal bleeding or epigastric pain [11]. Liver metastasis can spontaneously rupture and produce hemoperitoneum as they are highly vascular. Chemotherapy with EP for 1–3 weeks followed by EMA-EP can be given for such patients. Though they respond to chemotherapy, drug resistance is sometimes a challenge especially if the interval from antecedent pregnancy is long. Residual drug-resistant disease may be resected if feasible.

In cases of **liver metastasis** with or without metastasis in the brain, EMA-EP is preferred with dose escalation of Methotrexate to 1 gm/m^2 if the brain is involved, though there are different dose modifications [6]. Granulocyte colony-stimulating factors (GCSF) should be used to minimise myelosuppression, so that treatment delay can be avoided.

When **lung(s)** is involved with multiple metastases, the patient does have respiratory distress with associated haemoptysis and chest pain. The management of such cases is crucial with oxygen support, maybe in ICU with ventilatory support. One should be careful in providing ventilatory support to such patients. Positive pressure of ventilation may incite more pulmonary haemorrhage due to the friability of highly vascular tumour deposits inside the lungs. In such situations, early extubation with head down position can drain the collected blood [6]. Positive pressure ventilation at low pressure is the crux to prevent haemorrhage. In ICU, these patients should be offered maximum care taking into account the good survival once they tide over this crisis.

10.2.1 Management of Bleeding from Other Areas

Patients of ultrahigh-risk GTN are susceptible to haemorrhage from other metastatic sites too. Risk is exaggerated if EMA-CO regimen is initiated in treatment. This can be avoided by starting with low-dose induction chemotherapy as stated earlier. Expectant management of bleeding episodes can be done with bed rest, Tranexamic acid, gentle packing of the vagina if bleeding is from vaginal metastases. Very rarely vascular embolisation may be required in uterine bleeding or bleeding from metastatic sites from the liver, spleen, kidney and GI tract. Serum hCG levels >10,00,000 miu/ml have high tumour volume and are at risk for tumour lysis syndrome. The risk can be reduced with adequate hydration, allopurinol or rasburicase and careful attention to the renal function and electrolytes should be given. Other potential causes of death include neutropenic sepsis after chemotherapy. However, this does not happen now a day with the availability of growth factors and appropriate antibiotic use.

Thrombosis or tumour embolism is a potential cause of death in very sick patients. Use of low molecular weight heparin can be planned along with other supportive measures with caution in the situation of probability of more haemorrhagic incidence due to increased vascularity of the metastatic disease.

Targeted therapy with checkpoint inhibitor like pembrolizumab has been tried by some authors in high-risk/resistant GTN with favourable results [12].

A number of recent studies have confirmed the relatively poor survival statistics for these patients with cure rates of approximately 60–65% reported [3, 13]. Patients of ultrahigh-risk GTN do experience drug resistance to conventional therapy, mostly when associated with liver, brain and lung metastases. Once detected, by hCG monitoring, second-line CT with EP-EMA or TE/TP should be started. This will prevent drug resistance. The early deaths have dramatically reduced from the late 1990s due to the availability of expert service and also due to low-dose induction chemo with weekly cisplatin and etoposide for 1–3 weeks before starting on regular chemo, which results in a gradual reduction in tumour volume, thus avoiding complications like tumour lysis syndrome and haemorrhage. EP induction can be given for patients with >6 metastasis, HCG > 700,000 and FIGO score > 12 [14]. Ultrahigh-risk GTN is associated with a higher frequency of resistance to frontline chemotherapy especially with liver, brain metastasis and patients with long intervals from antecedent pregnancy. Resistance to chemotherapy was observed to be higher in frontline EMA-CO regimen than induction chemotherapy followed by EMA-CO (41 versus 28%, respectively) [15]. Regular monitoring with serum hCG helps to detect drug resistance and early switch to cisplatin-based therapy with EP-EMA or TP/TE will prevent the development of drug resistance. In selected cases, salvage surgery can be done. Though EMA-CO is the choice in high-risk cases, low-dose etoposide 100 mg/m^2 and ciplatin 20 mg/m^2 on D1 and 2 of every week for 1–3 weeks should be given to reduce tumour volume. Once the high-risk period is over and the patient is stabilised, EP-EMA can be started.

10.2.2 Follow-Up

The follow-up schedule is almost similar to that of other high-risk GTN. After normalisation of β-hCG levels, weekly estimation of β-hCG to be done until they are normal for three consecutive weeks, then monthly for 2 years. The patient should be followed up for at least 5 years. It is observed that the recurrence of GTN after 7 years of follow-up with normal findings is rare [16].

10.2.3 Prognosis

In a retrospective study of 143 cases of ultrahigh-risk patients by Yujia et al., it was found that complete remission could be achieved in 94 (65.7%) patients, and 15 (15.9%) patients experienced relapse after complete response. Their first-line chemotherapy was FAEV regimen (floxuridine, actinomycin-D, etoposide, vincristine). However, they have used EMA-CO, EMA-EP, TE/TP, etc. in case of failure or recurrence with their first-line CT. The 5-year overall survival in their study was 67.9% [17]. Moreover, interval since antecedent pregnancy plays a great role in prognostication. Disease occurrence after 2.8 years of the last pregnancy event has been taken as a worse prognostic index. The 5-year overall survival was 62.0% when the disease was diagnosed 2.8 years after the pregnancy event versus 94% in cases when the disease was diagnosed before 2.8 years. Survival is around 70–90% considering the site of disease, duration of last pregnancy and management intensity [5].

10.3 Summary and Conclusion

- Ultrahigh-risk GTN is a rare disease and presents management challenges.
- Once suspected/detected, should be shifted to tertiary centre or centres with expertise.
- Thorough counselling about the high morbidity, mortality, drug resistance and multi-specialty involvement, etc. should be done and consent to be taken.
- Ventilatory support may be deleterious in patients with massive lung disease—as positive pressure ventilation may cause more haemorrhage due to friable vascular tumour. Low-pressure ventilation and early extubation is advisable.
- Keeping in mind drug resistance (about one-third will develop drug resistance to Etoposide and Methotrexate based regimen), prompt switch over to second-line CT should be done.
- Granulocyte colony-stimulating factors (GCSF) should routinely be used to avoid delay in treatment.
- With all measures taken, 5% will die from the disease.
- Checkpoint inhibitors like pembrolizumab may be the future drugs in resistant GTN.
- Central database is the call for today for judicious management of the disease.

Management Algorithm of Ultrahigh-Risk GTN

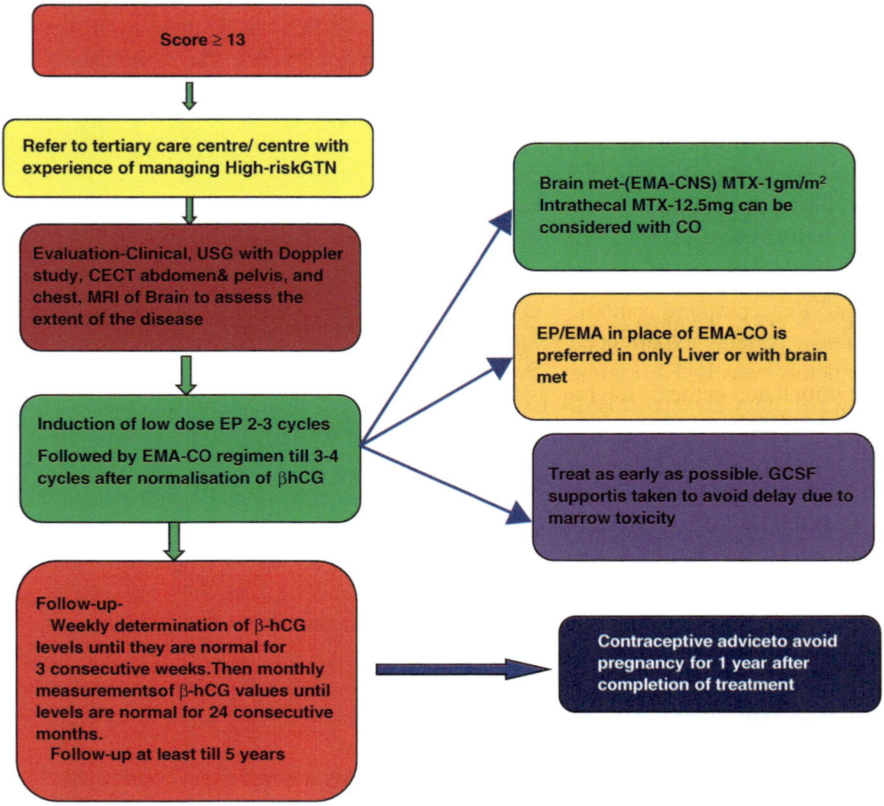

References

1. Lurain JR. Gestational trophoblastic disease II: classification and management of gestational trophoblastic neoplasia. Am J Obstet Gynecol. 2011;204:11–8.
2. Ngan HY, Seckl MJ, Berkowitz SR, Xiang Y, Sekharan PK, et al. "Update on the diagnosis and management of gestational trophoblastic disease." FIGO cancer report 2018. Int J Gynecol Obstet. 2018;143(Suppl. 2):79–85.
3. Bolze PA, Riedl C, Massardier J, et al. Mortality rate of gestational trophoblastic neoplasia with a FIGO score of ≥13. Am J Obstet Gynecol. 2016;214(3):390.e1–390.e8.
4. Abu-Rustum NR, Yashar CM, Bean S, et al. Gestational trophoblastic neoplasia, version 2.2019, NCCN clinical practice guidelines in oncology. J Natl Compr Cancer Netw. 2019;17:1374–91.
5. Coleman ER, Seckl JM. Ultra high risk GTN: what is it and how should we manage it? In: Hancock BW, Sekel MJ, Berkowitz RS, editors. Gestational trophoblastic disease. 4th ed; 2015. Chapter 18. p. 1–12.

6. Froeling FEM, Seckl MJ. Ultra high risk gestational trophoblastic neoplasia. TB Gyn Oncol. 2018:1016–20.
7. Alifrangis C, et al. EMA/CO for high-risk gestational trophoblastic neoplasia: good outcomes with induction low-dose etoposide-cisplatin and genetic analysis. J Clin Oncol. 2013;31(2):280–6.
8. Newlands ES, et al. Management of brain metastases in patients with high-risk gestational trophoblastic tumors. J Reprod Med. 2002;47(6):465–71.
9. Xiao C, et al. Management and prognosis of patients with brain metastasis from gestational trophoblastic neoplasia: a 24-year experience in Peking union medical college hospital. BMC Cancer. 2015;15:318.
10. Savage P, Kelpanides I, Tuthill M, et al. Brain metastases in gestational trophoblastic neoplasia: an update on incidence, management and outcome. Gynecol Oncol. 2015;137(1):73–6.
11. Bakri YN, Subhi J, Amer M, et al. Liver metastases of gestational trophoblastic tumor. Gynecol Oncol. 1993;48:110–3.
12. Gold AJ, Dioni G, Mariani A, Langstraat LC. A case of multi-agent drug resistant choriocarcinoma treated with Pembrolizumab. Gynecol Oncol Rep. 2020;32:100574. https://doi.org/10.1016/j.gore.2020.100574.
13. Kong Y, Yang J, Jiang F, et al. Clinical characteristics and prognosis of ultra high-risk gestational trophoblastic neoplasia patients: a retrospective cohort study. Gynecol Oncol. 2017;146:81–6.
14. Alifrangis C, Agarwal R, Short D, et al. EMA/CO for high risk gestational trophoblastic neoplasia: good outcomes with induction low-dose etoposide cisplatin at genetic analysis. J Clin Oncol. 2013;31:280–6.
15. Patel SM, Arora R, Tiwari R, Poddar P, Desai A, Mankad MH, et al. Management of "ultra-high risk" gestational trophoblastic neoplasia at a tertiary center in India. Ind J Med Paediatr Oncol. 2020;41:345–50.
16. Balachandran K, Salawu A, Ghorani E, Kaur B, Sebire NJ, Short D, et al. When to stop human chorionic gonadotrophin (hCG) surveillance after treatment with chemotherapy for gestational trophoblastic neoplasia (GTN): a national analysis on over 4,000 patients. Gynecol Oncol. 2019;155(1):8–12.
17. Yujia K, Junjun Y, Fang J, Jun Z, et al. Clinical characteristics and prognosis of ultra high-risk gestational trophoblastic neoplasia patients: a retrospective cohort study. Gynecol Oncol. 2017;146(1):81–86. https://doi.org/10.1016/j.ygyno.2017.04.010.

The Dynamic Scoring System and Staging

11

James R. Bentley

11.1 Historical Perspective

Currently, staging rules for gestational trophoblastic neoplasia follow the guidelines that were published in 2002, these constitute the 2000 FIGO Staging guidelines that were ratified in 2000 at the congress in Washington DC [1]. Prior to this time, there had been some anatomical staging per FIGO and other scoring systems developed and used in different parts of the world to aid management. The works behind these were done in several centers. Bagshawe in 1976 devised criteria that were developed based on a cohort of 300 and 17 patients treated at the Charing Cross Hospital from 1957 to 1973 [2]. This thus encompassed a time when chemotherapy was evolving significantly, with imaging and biochemical testing modalities being limited. The prognostic factors included age, parity, antecedent pregnancy, histological diagnosis, the interval from the antecedent pregnancy to chemotherapy starting, the hCG level, the ABO blood group, the extent of mononuclear infiltrates, and the size and site of metastases (Table 11.1). The women were divided into three groups depending on whether they were likely to be placed in remission by single agent chemotherapy, dual agent, or multi-agent regimens. This then morphed into the WHO scoring system that was used prior to 2002. In the United States, Hammond et al. evaluated the response to therapy in 91 patients treated at the Southeastern Regional Trophoblastic Disease Center [3]. They developed a system that placed people into high- and low-risk criteria and this was widely adopted (Table 11.2).

J. R. Bentley (✉)
Department of Obstetrics and Gynecology, Dalhousie University, Halifax, NS, Canada
e-mail: jim.bentley@dal.ca

B. Nayak, U. Singh (eds.), *Gestational Trophoblastic Disease*,
https://doi.org/10.1007/978-981-33-4878-3_11

Table 11.1 Bagshawe's prognostic scoring system for GTD (1976)

Score	0	10	20	40
Age (years)	<39	>39		
Parity	1,2,>4	3 or 4		
Antecedent pregnancy	Mole	Abortion	Term	
Histologic diagnosis (AP)	Invasive mole	Not known	Choriocarcinoma	
Interval (AP to start of chemo in months)	<4	4–7	7–12	>12
HCG (plasma IU/L or urine IU/day)	10^3–10^4	$<10^3$	10^4–10^5	$>10^5$
ABO groups (patient x husband)	A x A O or A x B O or A x AB	O x O A x O O x A B x B AN x B	B x O or A AB x O or A	
No. of metastases seen	None	1–4	4–8	>8
Site of metastases	Not detected Lungs Vagina	Spleen Kidney	Gastrointestinal tract Liver	Brain
Largest tumor mass diameter	3 cm	3–5 cm	5 cm	
Lymphocytic infiltration of tumor	Marked	Moderate or unknown	Slight	
Immune status	Reactive	Unknown	Unreactive	
Relapse after previous chemotherapy			Yes	

< 80 low risk, 80–120 medium risk, > 120 high risk

Table 11.2 Hammond's Southeastern Trophoblastic Disease Center Clinical Classification for GTD

I. Non-metastatic GTD
II. Metastatic GTD
A. Good prognosis
1. Urinary hCG <100,000 IU/24 h urine or < 40,000 IU/L serum
2. Symptoms present for less than 4 months
3. No brain or liver metastases
4. No prior chemotherapy
5. Pregnancy event is not term delivery (i.e., mole, ectopic, or spontaneous abortion)
B. Poor prognosis
1. Urinary hCG >100,000 IU/24 h urine or > 40,000 IU/L serum
2. Symptoms present for more than 4 months
3. Brain or liver metastases
4. Prior chemotherapy failure
5. Antecedent term pregnancy

11.2 Current Staging

The FIGO committee came together in 2000 and, after some discussion, brought together these prognostic scoring systems and anatomical-based scoring systems together to make the FIGO 2000 staging. This is dealt with in detail in the previous chapter (Tables 11.3 and 11.4).

The scoring system allows patients to be divided up into risk groups and it has long been suggested that there is a low-risk group of 0–6 and a high-risk group of seven or higher. There does remain some controversy in that women with a score of 5 or 6 seldom respond to single agent chemotherapy.

The format for reporting suggests that the FIGO anatomical stage be defined by a Roman numeral I, II, III, and IV and the actual risk be expressed by a number. For example, a 25-year-old patient with a rise in hCG to 1100 IU/ml at 6 weeks post evacuation for a molar pregnancy and disease confined to the uterus would be stage I:1, whereas a patient 35 years old post-term pregnancy with five lung metastases on a chest X-ray the largest of which is 2.5 cm and an hCG of 90,000 IU/ml would have a stage of III:8. The criteria for the diagnosis of post-hydatidiform mole were initially stated to include four criteria. Over recent years, the inclusion of diagnosing GTN when the hCG level remains elevated for over 6 months has been dropped by most authorities and no longer is on the 2018 FIGO update [4]. The first criteria is a plateau of hCG over a period of 3 weeks or longer with four measurements, i.e., days 1, 7, 14, and 21. The plateau is defined as less than a 10% change in values.

Table 11.3 FIGO 2000 staging of GTN

Stage I	Disease confined to the uterus
Stage II	GTN extends outside the uterus but is confined to the genital structures (adnexa, vagina, broad ligament)
Stage III	GTN extends to the lungs with or without genital tract involvement
Stage IV	All other metastatic sites

Table 11.4 FIGO/WHO scoring system

WHO risk factor score	0	1	2	4
Age	<40	>40		
Antecedent pregnancy	Mole	Abortion	Term	
Interval from index pregnancy, months	<4	4–6	7–12	>12
Pretreatment hCG, mIU/ml	$<10^3$	$>10^3$–10^4	$>10^4$–10^5	$>10^5$
Largest tumor size including uterus, cm	–	3–4	≥5	–
Site of metastases	Lung	Spleen, kidney	Gastrointestinal tract	Brain, liver
Number of metastases identified	–	1–4	5–8	>8
Previous failed chemotherapy			Single drug	Two or more drugs

The second is a rise in hCG over a period of 2 weeks or more and the third criteria are the histologic diagnosis of choriocarcinoma.

The 2018 update gives us contemporary guidelines around how to investigate patients who have trophoblastic neoplasia. A chest X-ray is appropriate to diagnose lung metastases and can be used for counting the number of lung metastases to evaluate the risk score. A chest CT may be used, but should not be used to count the number of metastases. Liver metastases can be diagnosed by ultrasound or CT scanning and an MRI or CT scan may be used for brain metastases.

More recently, the UK group did look at factors that could be used to simplify the scoring system. They did a multivariate analysis of 813 cases from 2003 to 2019. They evaluated which factors could be individually predictive of single agent drug resistance. The predictive factors were pretreatment hCG over 10,000 IU/ml, an interval exceeding 7 months and tumor size over 5 cm. In a final risk model, they used age, pretreatment serum hCG, number of metastases, antecedent pregnancy, and interval, which had a very high concordance with the FIGO 2000 system [5].

11.3 Dynamic Scoring System

Dr. Kohorn from Yale University, USA, has recommended that the scoring and risk factor analysis be modified and that a dynamic system be used [6].

It has been suggested that, for completeness, a diagnosis of hydatidiform mole should be included as stage 0 in the FIGO staging. Currently, it is noted that currently there are no stage 0's in gynecological cancer for any tumor site. For a hydatidiform mole of either partial or complete, it has been suggested that this would be stage 0 when diagnosed post evacuation and you could add a "c" to indicate complete or "p" to indicate partial. The subclassification should only be noted if there is immunohistochemistry with p57 or DNA ploidy confirmation of partial mole. This is because of the challenges with accurately diagnosing partial moles in early pregnancy. After the stage 0, the FIGO prognostic score is added. There are risk factors such as very high hCG, theca-luteal cysts, and uterine size that could be added to this stage 0 as they do provide some modification of risk to the patient. Despite this being suggested in 2007 there has been little adoption of this in reports or the literature.

Dr. Kohorn also has tried to address the issue of invasive mole. This is clinically not commonly diagnosed in North America or Europe; however, in other areas, patients may present with massive intra-abdominal bleeding due to penetration of the uterus by gestational trophoblastic disease. The histology may be of an invasive mole or potentially of a choriocarcinoma. He raised the issue of whether this should be classified as a separate entity or subclassified within GTN. He suggested that this be classified as a stage 1 GTN with the degree of myometrial invasion by imaging being described by an M and using 0 for myometrial invasion, S for superficial invasion, I for intermediate invasion, and F for full myometrial invasion. We then would add a note for pathology with M indicating mole histology, while CH would indicate choriocarcinoma. This has the potential to describe a patient who presents with a post full-term pregnancy with hematoperitoneum and full penetration and a pathology showing choriocarcinoma to be described as: I:m.F.CH.

When we stage a patient, we traditionally use the initial staging and do not change the stage as the patient progresses through either cure or relapse. Dr. Kohorn had suggested the introduction of a dynamic staging system for gestational trophoblastic disease. This would retain the initial stage and, if there is a progression, this can be recorded. It is generally accepted that the patient will be scored before treatment is initiated or when there is a change in treatment.

For example, a 28-year-old lady presents with PV bleeding, has an hCG of 150,000 IU/ml, has an evacuation, and pathology confirms a complete hydatidiform mole. In the suggested terminology this would be stage 0c. She is then followed with serum hCG testing and this rises at 4 months to a value of 1350 IU/ml. Subsequent investigations show three 1-cm metastases on chest X-ray with ten more of a smaller size on a CT scan. Imaging of the head and abdomen are negative. She would be scored at this time as FIGO stage III:3. The patient is treated with a single agent methotrexate and after an initial drop has a rise in hcG 10 months later to 700 IU/ml. The patient is reimaged and in addition to 5 lung metastases on CXR has a liver lesion measuring 3 cm. She would now be stage IV:9. This progression can be noted as Oc:1 > III:3 > IV:9.

11.4 Conclusion

After evaluating the literature on this, I cannot find widespread recognition or need for use of a complicated dynamics staging system. It does, however, raise the issue and allowing the patient to be re-staged throughout the course of treatment does give information. I do not fully support the use of a stage 0 or stage I to define the molar pregnancy and invasive mole. Simple descriptive terms are adequate to describe these findings.

The main aim of any classification and staging system is to ensure that we all speak the same language and describe our patients adequately, with a secondary note that it might help direct care. Certainly, the FIGO 2000 staging system has achieved a uniform approach internationally and, at this stage, there are minor changes that could be considered. I do feel that a simple dynamic system that allows you to describe how a patient goes from stage-to-stage in complex situations would be beneficial.

References

1. Ngan HY, Bender H, Benedet JL, Jones H, Montruccoli GC, Pecorelli S, et al. Gestational trophoblastic neoplasia, FIGO 2000 staging and classification. Int J Gynaecol Obstet. 2003;83(Suppl 1):175–7.
2. Bagshawe KD. Risk and prognostic factors in trophoblastic neoplasia. Cancer. 1976;38:1373–85.
3. Hammond CB, Borchert LG, Tyrewy L, et al. Treatment of metastatic trophoblastic disease: good and poor prognosis. Am. J. Obstet Gynecol. 1973;115:451–7.

4. Ngan HY, Seckl MJ, Berkowitz RS, a. Update on the diagnosis and management of gestational trophoblastic disease. Inj J Gynecol Obstet. 2018;143(Suppl 2):79–85.
5. Eysbouts YK, Ottevanger PB, Massuger LFAG, et al. Can the FIGO 2000 scoring system for gestational trophoblastic neoplasia be simplified? A new retrospective analysis from a nationwide dataset. Ann Oncol. 2017;28(8):1856–61.
6. Kohorn EI. Dynamic staging and risk factor scoring for gestational trophoblastic disease. Int J Gynecol Cancer. 2007;17:1124–30.

Surgical Management of Gestational Trophoblastic Disease

12

Saketh R. Guntupalli and Marisa R. Moroney

12.1 Introduction

Gestational trophoblastic disease (GTD) is a spectrum of premalignant and malignant tumors that develop from placental tissue and thus are associated with pregnancy. GTD includes complete and partial hydatidiform mole, invasive mole, choriocarcinoma, atypical placental site nodule (APSN), placental site trophoblastic tumor (PSTT), and epithelioid trophoblastic tumor (ETT). The malignant GTD entities (invasive mole, choriocarcinoma, PSTT, and ETT) are collectively termed gestational trophoblastic neoplasia (GTN) and have the ability to invade and metastasize [1–4]. Outcomes for GTD have significantly improved over the last few decades with overall cure rates now well over 90%. These improved outcomes are due to utilization of the tumor marker human chorionic gonadotropin (hCG) for disease diagnosis and monitoring, clinical risk-stratification and treatment individualization based on well-defined prognostic factors, increased referral to or consultation with disease specialists, development of improved chemotherapy regimens, and the use of combined treatment modalities (chemotherapy, surgery, radiation) for high-risk patients [1, 4–8].

Chemotherapy is essential to the treatment of GTN and a key factor in the improved cure rates. Although surgery is not as frequently indicated or utilized in the management of GTD, there are key instances in which surgery plays an important role in improving patient outcomes. These instances include primary uterine evacuation of hydatidiform moles, primary hysterectomy for molar pregnancies and

S. R. Guntupalli (✉) · M. R. Moroney
Department of Obstetrics and Gynecology, Division of Gynecologic Oncology, University of Colorado School of Medicine, Aurora, CO, USA
e-mail: saketh.guntupalli@ucdenver.edu

B. Nayak, U. Singh (eds.), *Gestational Trophoblastic Disease*,
https://doi.org/10.1007/978-981-33-4878-3_12

malignant GTN, secondary hysterectomy and/or other excisional procedures for chemotherapy-resistant disease, excisional procedures to improve chemotherapy response, and surgical management of disease complications [1, 4–7]. In this chapter, we will review in detail the indications for surgery in the management of GTD.

12.2 Hydatidiform Mole

Standard treatment for hydatidiform moles, or molar pregnancies, consists of uterine evacuation and subsequent close surveillance of serum hCG levels. The uterine evacuation provides the primary treatment through removal of the molar pregnancy, while also allowing for diagnostic pathologic and genetic evaluation. Serial serum hCG levels are then performed in order to confirm resolution of the molar pregnancy and monitor for the development of post-molar GTN [1, 3, 4, 6–9]. Surgery, in the form of uterine evacuation, thus plays an essential role in the management of molar pregnancies.

12.2.1 Dilation and Suction Curettage

The preferred surgical method for uterine evacuation of a molar pregnancy in a patient who desires to maintain her fertility is dilation and suction curettage (D&C). Suction curettage has low complication rates, high efficacy in achieving complete uterine evacuation, and low risk of post-molar GTN [3, 4, 6, 9]. Prior to performing the suction curettage, a patient should have a complete preoperative work-up evaluating for anemia, thyroid disorder, liver or kidney dysfunction, cardiac abnormalities, and preeclampsia. A serum hCG should be collected as part of the patient's continued monitoring for disease resolution versus the development of post-molar GTN [3, 8, 9]. Preoperatively, a blood type and antibody screen should also be performed both because of the risk of hemorrhage and in order to evaluate for need for Rh immune globulin. RhD antigen is present in trophoblasts, and therefore all patients with an Rh-negative blood type should receive Rh-immune globulin at the time of uterine evacuation [1, 3, 8, 9].

Once in an operating room with effective anesthesia, the D&C procedure is started by dilating the cervix with Hegar or Pratt dilators to allow for a large suction cannula, usually 12–14 mm. The suction cannula is then introduced into the uterus and gently rotated to remove the uterine contents and begin uterine involution [3, 6]. Once the cervix is dilated and suction curettage is initiated, intravenous (IV) oxytocin is usually infused in order to assist with uterine involution and contractility. Bimanual massage and other uterotonics (prostaglandins and methylergonovine) can also be utilized to assist with uterine involution [1, 3, 4, 6]. Following suction curettage, a gentle sharp curettage is performed in order to ensure complete uterine evaluation [3, 6]. Care is taken to avoid aggressive sharp curettage, as it carries a risk of development of uterine synechiae and Asherman's syndrome [6]. The entire

D&C procedure can be done under ultrasound guidance in order to decrease the risk of uterine perforation and ensure complete removal of uterine contents [1, 4, 6].

As previously mentioned, one of the main reasons that suction curettage is a preferred method for uterine evacuation of a molar pregnancy is its low complication rate. Uterine perforation is a rare complication that occurs in less than 1% of suction curettage procedures performed for evacuation of a molar pregnancy [6, 10]. When a uterine perforation occurs, all instruments should be removed from the uterus (suction cannula or sharp curette) immediately and oxytocin infusion rates should be increased. Laparoscopy or a laparotomy should then be performed to evaluate the perforation site on the uterus and to evaluate for any injury to intra-abdominal structures, specifically the bowl. If the perforation site is hemostatic and there is no intra-abdominal injury, sharp curettage can be completed under direct visualization and no repair of the perforation site is required. If there is active bleeding at the perforation site, repair should be attempted in an individualized manner; however, a hysterectomy may be required [6].

There is an increased risk for complications at the time of uterine evacuation in patients who present with uterine size greater than 16 weeks' gestation, specifically increased risk of uterine perforation, hemorrhage, and pulmonary complications [3, 4, 6]. Suction curettage is still the preferred method of uterine evacuation in these patients, if they desire to maintain their fertility. Because of the increased complication risk in these patients, preoperative evaluation and preparation should include (in addition to standard preoperative management as described above) a crossmatch for two units of blood and two large-bore IV catheters. Intraoperatively, these patients should have close monitoring and judicious fluid repletion in order to decrease rates of pulmonary complications. Fortunately, the incidence of uterine enlargement greater than 16 weeks' gestation in molar pregnancy is decreasing, likely due to increased utilization of early ultrasound in pregnancy [3, 6].

12.2.2 Other Forms of Fertility-Sparing Uterine Evacuation

Historically, prior to the widespread availability and use of suction curettage, induction of labor and hysterotomy were surgical techniques that were utilized for uterine evacuation of molar pregnancies. Both of these techniques are no longer recommended as they increase patient morbidity and risk of post-molar GTN. Both procedures are associated with an increased risk of blood loss and incomplete uterine evacuation, requiring subsequent dilation and suction curettage. Hysterotomy is an abdominal surgery and thus is associated with a longer postoperative recovery. The vertical incision made in the uterine myometrium during a hysterotomy also precludes the patient from future labor and thus commits them to cesarean section in future pregnancies. Multiple reviews have evaluated the risk of post-molar GTN and demonstrated that patients undergoing uterine evacuation by either induction of labor or hysterotomy have significantly higher rates of post-molar GTN compared to patients undergoing suction curettage for uterine evacuation [3, 6, 11, 12]. Again, for these reasons, suction curettage is the preferred method of uterine evacuation in patients who desire to maintain their fertility.

12.2.3 Hysterectomy

Primary hysterectomy is an alternative method for uterine evacuation in women who have completed childbearing [1, 3, 4, 6, 9]. Hysterectomy can be performed by any route—abdominal, laparoscopic, or robotic—depending on the standard surgical factors of uterine size and mobility, pelvic access, and patient co-morbidities. Primary hysterectomy as treatment for molar pregnancy has the advantages of complete evacuation of disease by removing the uterus, as well as sterilization in those patients that no longer desire to maintain their fertility [3, 6]. When performing a hysterectomy for management of molar pregnancy, the adnexa should not be removed, unless a patient has obvious metastatic disease to the adnexa. Even when theca lutein cysts are present, the adnexa do not need to be removed, as theca lutein cysts usually resolve spontaneously following uterine evacuation of the molar pregnancy [3, 6, 13].

Primary hysterectomy also decreases the risk of post-molar GTN compared with suction curettage. This is because, by removing the uterus, the risk of local myometrial invasion (i.e., an invasive mole) is eliminated. However, the risk of post-molar GTN is not completely resolved, as there remains a risk of metastatic disease. It is therefore important to continue postoperative surveillance of serial serum hCG levels in patients who have had primary hysterectomies for their molar pregnancy [3, 6, 9]. The risk of post-molar GTN following primary hysterectomy is approximately 3–5% versus an approximately 20% risk following suction curettage [3, 4, 6, 9, 12]. This risk reduction is especially relevant in older patients with molar pregnancies as older age is an independent risk factor for post-molar GTN. Multiple retrospective studies have specifically evaluated women over 40 years old with molar pregnancies and demonstrated that primary hysterectomy significantly decreases the risk of post-molar GTN compared to suction curettage [3, 6, 14–16].

12.3 Malignant GTN

Management of GTN is determined by the World Health Organization (WHO) scoring system, which is based on well-defined prognostic factors. For first-line therapy, low-risk patients (WHO score 0–6) are typically treated with single-agent chemotherapy (methotrexate or actinomycin D), while high-risk patients (WHO score ≥ 7) are typically treated with multi-agent chemotherapy (EMA/CO—etoposide, methotrexate, actinomycin D, cyclophosphamide, and vincristine). Chemotherapy is a mainstay in the management of GTN. Treatment with chemotherapy allows for the majority of patients to achieve cure while maintaining fertility. However, management is individualized based on factors like location of metastatic disease, chemotherapy-resistance, fertility desires, etc., and certain patients with GTN still benefit from surgical management [1, 4, 6, 7].

12.3.1 Second D&C

A second D&C can be considered in patients who have been diagnosed with post-molar GTN and are low-risk. This second D&C is performed via the same technique as described above for molar pregnancies. Observational and prospective studies have demonstrated that 40–68% of low-risk, non-metastatic GTN patients will be cured with a second D&C, and thus will be able to avoid chemotherapy. These studies also demonstrate that certain patient and disease factors increase the risk of needing subsequent chemotherapy including age less than 19 or greater than 40 and WHO score greater than 4. There is inconsistent evidence as to whether an elevated hCG above any certain numeric cutoff is predictive of response to second D&C [1, 17, 18].

12.3.2 Hysterectomy

Primary hysterectomy can also be considered in patients who have been diagnosed with non-metastatic, post-molar GTN, are low-risk, and have completed childbearing. Similarly to a second D&C, it has been demonstrated that hysterectomy in this low-risk, non-metastatic population can result in complete remission, thus allowing a patient to avoid chemotherapy [1, 6, 19]. For those patients that do require postoperative chemotherapy following a hysterectomy, studies have demonstrated that the hysterectomy may decrease the number of required chemotherapy cycles to achieve remission [6, 7, 20, 21]. In contrast, primary hysterectomy for patients with high-risk and metastatic GTN has been shown to have no benefit in terms of cure rates or number of required chemotherapy cycles, and therefore, primary hysterectomy should not be offered to these patients [6, 20].

A delayed hysterectomy can also improve patient outcomes in a select patient population. Multiple studies have demonstrated that patients with low-risk (WHO score 0–6), non-metastatic GTN that have demonstrated persistent disease, or chemotherapy-resistance, following primary treatment with single-agent chemotherapy, a delayed hysterectomy can result in complete remission in greater than 90% of patients. Therefore, delayed hysterectomy should be offered to patients with low-risk, non-metastatic, chemotherapy-resistant GTN in order to attempt to avoid subsequent multi-agent chemotherapy [6, 7, 19, 20]. Patients with low-risk and high-risk GTN with small quantity extra-uterine or metastatic disease who have recurrent or chemotherapy-resistant disease can also experience some benefit from a delayed hysterectomy. Multiple reviews have demonstrated that over 75% of patients in this population can achieve complete remission with delayed hysterectomy. However, achieving remission in this setting is highly dependent on disease burden; patients with large-volume disseminated disease are less likely to receive benefit from hysterectomy as their tumor burden is more extensive [6, 7, 22–24]. Finally, hysterectomy is indicated in patients who have GTN and significant, life-threatening uterine hemorrhage. In these cases, hysterectomy improves clinical outcomes by resulting in the cessation of bleeding. Another treatment modality that can be considered to manage life-threatening uterine hemorrhage is uterine artery embolization [4, 7, 19, 23].

In contrast to invasive mole and choriocarcinoma, PSTT and ETT are relatively chemotherapy-resistant and thus surgery, specifically hysterectomy, plays a much larger role in their management. For non-metastatic PSTT and ETT, primary hysterectomy is the recommended first-line therapy. Over 66% of patients with non-metastatic PSTT and ETT can achieve complete remission with primary hysterectomy alone. Due to the tendency toward chemotherapy resistance, surgical debulking consisting of hysterectomy, lymphadenectomy and excision of metastatic disease are recommended with concomitant chemotherapy for patients with metastatic PSTT and ETT [1, 6, 7, 25–27].

Hysterectomy is usually performed through an abdominal route for patients with GTN, as it allows for full abdominal exploration for metastatic disease. Laparoscopic-assisted vaginal hysterectomy has been reported in the literature and does allow for abdominal evaluation through laparoscopy, as would a total laparoscopic hysterectomy or a robotic hysterectomy. Minimally invasive hysterectomies would also have the benefit of shorter postoperative recovery [6, 28]. The hysterectomy should include the removal of the uterus and cervix. Radical hysterectomies, or types II and III hysterectomies, involving the removal of larger portions of the parametria, uterine vasculature, uterosacral ligament, and vagina have also been reported in the literature and may be indicated to achieve full resection of disease [6, 22, 25]. Oophorectomy does not need to be performed as GTN rarely metastasizes to the ovaries and is not a hormonally driven malignancy [6, 20, 29]. Though the ovaries look cystic they should be saved as the cysts regress over time.

12.3.3 Myometrial Resection

Myometrial resection for conservative, fertility-sparing management can be considered in very select patients with low-risk, non-metastatic GTN [4, 6, 25]. Myometrial resection with uterine repair has been studied in patients with invasive mole and PSTT. Studies have shown that patients with non-metastatic invasive moles can achieve complete remission following myometrial resection but may require subsequent chemotherapy in order to do so. These patients with invasive moles treated via myometrial resection have also been shown to have similar subsequent pregnancy rates as patients with invasive moles treated with chemotherapy alone. Therefore, chemotherapy as first-line therapy and myometrial resection for salvage therapy could be considered [6, 30, 31]. A small number of cases of PSTT treated with myometrial resection have been reported in the literature and many of these cases have required subsequent completion of hysterectomy due to persistent, unresected uterine disease [6, 25, 32–34]. Due to the rarity of ETT, the role of myometrial resection in the management of ETT is unproven [25]. In patients with low-risk, non-metastatic GTN who have an indication for surgical management but strongly desire fertility preservation, counseling needs to be performed on the increased safety and efficacy of hysterectomy over myometrial resection. They also need to be counseled on the risk of persistent, unresected uterine disease requiring the need for completion hysterectomy. In order to select appropriate patients for myometrial resection and decrease the risk of persistent, unresected uterine disease, these patients should have an extensive preoperative evaluation including pelvic ultrasound with doppler flow and magnetic resonance imaging [6, 25].

12.3.4 Surgical Excision of Metastatic GTN

Pulmonary resection via thoracotomy or video-assisted thoracoscopic surgery is the most common surgery performed for excision of metastatic GTN lesions and is an important component of the management of high-risk, chemotherapy-resistant GTN [6, 35]. Pulmonary resection is most frequently performed in patients with recurrent, chemotherapy-resistant lesions, and over 70% cure rate has been reported. The patients that are the most likely to benefit and achieve complete remission are those that have isolated, unilateral pulmonary lesions and low hCG levels. Prior to performing pulmonary resection, full-body imaging should be utilized to evaluate for other locations of metastatic disease [4, 6, 7, 35, 36].

Craniotomy for resection of metastatic brain lesions is another excision procedure performed in patients with high-risk metastatic GTN. However, due to the poor prognosis associated with brain metastases from GTN, the utilization of brain irradiation to treat brain metastases, and the risks associated with craniotomy, it is much less commonly used compared to pulmonary resection. Craniotomy has been demonstrated to be most successful in treating brain metastases from GTN in patients with isolated, peripheral lesions and in combination with chemotherapy and/or brain irradiation. Craniotomy is also indicated for decompression in patients with high-risk GTN who have brain metastases and neurologic deterioration due to hemorrhage and increasing intercranial pressure [6, 7, 37, 38].

Vaginal metastases from GTN tend to be highly vascular and therefore should typically not be biopsied or excised. If bleeding from vaginal metastases is occurring, possible treatment modalities include vaginal packing, irradiation, and selective artery embolization. In an attempt to achieve disease remission, vaginal metastases are often treated with chemotherapy [6]. Other possible metastatic disease sites from GTN include the kidneys, the GI tract, and the liver. Often metastases to these sites occur with extensive dissemination of disease and thus are treated with chemotherapy. However, as in pulmonary and brain metastases, surgical excision can help to achieve complete remission in the setting of isolated, chemotherapy-resistant lesions [4, 6, 7].

References

1. Abu-Rustum NR, et al. Gestational trophoblastic neoplasia, version 2.2019, NCCN clinical practice guidelines in oncology. J Natl Compr Cancer Netw. 2019;17(11):1374–91.
2. Berek JS, Hacker NF. Berek & Hacker's gynecologic oncology. 6th ed. Philadelphia: Wolters Kluwer; 2015. p. xvi. 960 pages
3. Lurain JR. Gestational trophoblastic disease I: epidemiology, pathology, clinical presentation and diagnosis of gestational trophoblastic disease, and management of hydatidiform mole. Am J Obstet Gynecol. 2010;203(6):531–9.
4. Ngan HYS, et al. Update on the diagnosis and management of gestational trophoblastic disease. Int J Gynaecol Obstet. 2018;143(Suppl 2):79–85.
5. Brown J, et al. 15 years of progress in gestational trophoblastic disease: scoring, standardization, and salvage. Gynecol Oncol. 2017;144(1):200–7.
6. Doll KM, Soper JT. The role of surgery in the management of gestational trophoblastic neoplasia. Obstet Gynecol Surv. 2013;68(7):533–42.
7. Lurain JR. Gestational trophoblastic disease II: classification and management of gestational trophoblastic neoplasia. Am J Obstet Gynecol. 2011;204(1):11–8.
8. Soper JT. Gestational trophoblastic neoplasia. Curr Opin Obstet Gynecol. 1990;2(1):92–7.
9. Berkowitz RS, Goldstein DP. Clinical practice. Molar pregnancy. N Engl J Med. 2009;360(16):1639–45.
10. Mungan T, et al. Hydatidiform mole: clinical analysis of 310 patients. Int J Gynaecol Obstet. 1996;52(3):233–6.
11. Tidy JA, et al. Gestational trophoblastic disease: a study of mode of evacuation and subsequent need for treatment with chemotherapy. Gynecol Oncol. 2000;78(3 Pt 1):309–12.
12. Curry SL, et al. Hydatidiform mole: diagnosis, management, and long-term followup of 347 patients. Obstet Gynecol. 1975;45(1):1–8.
13. Montz FJ, Schlaerth JB, Morrow CP. The natural history of theca lutein cysts. Obstet Gynecol. 1988;72(2):247–51.
14. Zhao P, Chen Q, Lu W. Comparison of different therapeutic strategies for complete hydatidiform mole in women at least 40 years old: a retrospective cohort study. BMC Cancer. 2017;17(1):733.
15. Elias KM, Goldstein DP, Berkowitz RS. Complete hydatidiform mole in women older than age 50. J Reprod Med. 2010;55(5–6):208–12.
16. Elias KM, et al. Complete hydatidiform mole in women aged 40 to 49 years. J Reprod Med. 2012;57(5–6):254–8.
17. Osborne RJ, et al. Second curettage for low-risk nonmetastatic gestational trophoblastic neoplasia. Obstet Gynecol. 2016;128(3):535–42.
18. Pezeshki M, et al. The role of repeat uterine evacuation in the management of persistent gestational trophoblastic disease. Gynecol Oncol. 2004;95(3):423–9.
19. Eysbouts YK, et al. The added value of hysterectomy in the management of gestational trophoblastic neoplasia. Gynecol Oncol. 2017;145(3):536–42.
20. Hammond CB, Weed JC Jr, Currie JL. The role of operation in the current therapy of gestational trophoblastic disease. Am J Obstet Gynecol. 1980;136(7):844–58.
21. Suzuka K, et al. Adjuvant hysterectomy in low-risk gestational trophoblastic disease. Obstet Gynecol. 2001;97(3):431–4.
22. Doumplis D, et al. A review of the management by hysterectomy of 25 cases of gestational trophoblastic tumours from March 1993 to January 2006. BJOG. 2007;114(9):1168–71.
23. Fang J, et al. Role of adjuvant hysterectomy in management of high-risk gestational trophoblastic neoplasia. Int J Gynecol Cancer. 2012;22(3):509–14.
24. Mutch DG, et al. Recurrent gestational trophoblastic disease. Experience of the Southeastern Regional Trophoblastic Disease Center. Cancer. 1990;66(5):978–82.

25. Gadducci A, et al. Placental site trophoblastic tumor and epithelioid trophoblastic tumor: clinical and pathological features, prognostic variables and treatment strategy. Gynecol Oncol. 2019;153(3):684–93.
26. Papadopoulos AJ, et al. Twenty-five years' clinical experience with placental site trophoblastic tumors. J Reprod Med. 2002;47(6):460–4.
27. Sobecki-Rausch J, et al. Surgery and platinum/etoposide-based chemotherapy for the treatment of epithelioid trophoblastic tumor. Int J Gynecol Cancer. 2018;28(6):1117–22.
28. Lang JF, Childers JM, Surwit EA. Laparoscopic hysterectomy for persistent gestational trophoblastic neoplasia. J Am Assoc Gynecol Laparosc. 1995;2(4):475–7.
29. Berkowitz BJ, et al. Ovarian conservation in placental site trophoblastic tumor. Gynecol Oncol. 1990;37(2):239–43.
30. Case AM, et al. Fertility-sparing surgery, with subsequent pregnancy, in persistent gestational trophoblastic neoplasia: case report. Hum Reprod. 2001;16(2):360–4.
31. Kanazawa K, et al. Clinical evaluation of focal excision of myometrial lesion for treatment of invasive hydatidiform mole. Acta Obstet Gynecol Scand. 1988;67(6):487–92.
32. Pfeffer PE, et al. Fertility-sparing partial hysterectomy for placental-site trophoblastic tumour. Lancet Oncol. 2007;8(8):744–6.
33. Saso S, et al. Placental site trophoblastic tumours and the concept of fertility preservation. BJOG. 2012;119(3):369–74. discussion 374
34. Chiofalo B, et al. Fertility sparing strategies in patients affected by placental site trophoblastic tumor. Curr Treat Options in Oncol. 2017;18(10):58.
35. Kanis MJ, Lurain JR. Pulmonary resection in the management of high-risk gestational trophoblastic neoplasia. Int J Gynecol Cancer. 2016;26(4):796–800.
36. Tomoda Y, et al. Surgical indications for resection in pulmonary metastasis of choriocarcinoma. Cancer. 1980;46(12):2723–30.
37. Jr. Evans AC, et al. Gestational trophoblastic disease metastatic to the central nervous system. Gynecol Oncol. 1995;59(2):226–30.
38. Ishizuka T, et al. Intracranial metastasis of choriocarcinoma. A clinicopathologic study. Cancer. 1983;52(10):1896–903.

13 Placental Site and Epithelioid Trophoblastic Tumours: Rare Varieties of Gestational Trophoblastic Neoplasia

Shweta Tahlan, Vaishali Paliwal, and Amita Maheshwari

13.1 Introduction

Placental site trophoblastic tumours (PSTT) and epithelioid trophoblastic tumours (ETT) are rare varieties of gestational trophoblastic neoplasia (GTN); more common types are invasive mole and gestational choriocarcinoma. PSTT and ETT develop from the extravillous intermediate trophoblasts. They can follow normal pregnancy, abortion or molar pregnancy and are usually diagnosed months or years after the antecedent pregnancy. The exact incidence of these tumours is not known; however, it has been reported to be less than 1–3% of all GTN patients in various series [1–4]. The approximate number of reported cases in the literature are over 300 for PSTT and over 100 for ETT [5].

PSTT was first described by Kurman in 1976 as syncytial endometritis: *a benign lesion that stimulates malignant tumour* on histopathology and named it trophoblastic pseudotumour of the uterus [6]. In 1981, Scully and Young described the morphological details and recognised it as a neoplastic tumour, and coined the term PSTT [7]. In 1983, the World Health Organization (WHO) formally acknowledged the neoplastic nature of this lesion and adopted the terminology of PSTT. In 1998, Shih and Kurman described epithelioid trophoblastic tumours (ETT) as a separate trophoblastic tumour of malignant nature [8]. ETT has distinct morphologic features from PSTT but closely resembles its behaviour. It also simulates squamous cell carcinoma, making its diagnosis very challenging.

S. Tahlan · V. Paliwal · A. Maheshwari (✉)
Division of Gynecologic Oncology, Tata Memorial Centre & Homi Bhabha National Institute, Mumbai, India

B. Nayak, U. Singh (eds.), *Gestational Trophoblastic Disease*,
https://doi.org/10.1007/978-981-33-4878-3_13

13.2 Clinical Presentation

PSTT and ETT can develop after normal pregnancy (abortion or full term) or molar pregnancy. The presentation is usually months or years after the antecedent pregnancy event. The mean interval for PSTT is around 3 years [9], with a range from 2 to 5 years reported in a review [3], whereas the mean interval tends to be longer for ETT at around 6 years [10]. Rarely, these tumours can be found in peri- and postmenopausal women.

Typically, the patient presents with irregular vaginal bleeding long after a non-molar pregnancy [3, 9, 11]. There may be a history of amenorrhea as well. They can also present with symptoms of pelvic mass due to an enlarged uterus. About 16–54% cases of PSTT and 25–35% cases of ETT have metastatic disease at the time of diagnosis [2, 8, 11, 12]. The most common site of metastasis is the lung; others are the liver, bowel, lymph nodes, vagina, ovary, broad ligament, brain, kidney and spleen [2, 11, 13]. These tumours have a higher propensity for lymph node metastasis compared to other GTN [14]. There have been rare reports of other presentations like virilization, galactorrhea and nephrotic syndrome [5].

13.3 Diagnosis and Pre-treatment Evaluation

A high degree of suspicion is required to diagnose PSTT/ETT. A detailed obstetric history should be taken of all past pregnancy events. General physical examination along with complete pelvic examination should be done. Women in the reproductive age group presenting with metastatic disease with unknown primary or irregular vaginal bleeding should have hCG level measurement [15].

PSTT and ETT produce low levels of hCG unlike other GTN. A majority of patients have hCG value less than 1000 mU/ml [3, 9, 16]. PSTT/ETT should be suspected if the hCG level is low for the volume of disease seen on imaging. Measurement of the free beta subunit of hCG can also help us distinguishing PSTT from other GTDs, as the proportion of free beta subunit of hCG to total hCG is higher in these tumours [17].

Pelvic ultrasound is an excellent modality for the diagnosis of PSTT/ETT and also helps to assess tumour vascularity. Zhou et al. described three types of presentations on sonography. Type 1 consists of a heterogenous solid mass in the uterine cavity with mild to moderate vascularity. Type 2 consists of a solid mass in the myometrium with varying degree of vascularity. Type 3 consists of cystic lesions in the myometrium with a high degree of vascularity [18]. These findings can also help in planning the treatment; hypervascular tumours can be considered for selective embolization before a definitive surgical procedure.

In patients with ETT, transvaginal ultrasound (TVS) may show irregular anechoic lacunae in the myometrium, some filled with low resistance turbulent blood flow. On Doppler, typically a peripheral pattern of signals is seen, distinct from invasive mole and choriocarcinoma. These USG findings can help differentiate an ETT from other types of GTN [19].

Extensive staging investigations are required for women suspected to have PSTT/ ETT. These include contrast-enhanced CT scan of thorax and abdomen, MRI of brain and pelvis and a Doppler ultrasound of the pelvis [15]. PET CT is not recommended as an imaging modality for initial staging. It may be more helpful to assess sites for surgical resection in recurrent/relapsed disease [20].

A histopathological confirmation on tissue biopsy is essential for diagnosis [15]. These tumours can be confused with choriocarcinoma leading to delay in proper treatment including surgical intervention [13].

13.4 Pathology

Placental site trophoblastic tumours and epithelioid trophoblastic tumours develop from extravillous intermediate trophoblasts, in contrast to choriocarcinoma and invasive mole which develop from the villous trophoblasts (cytotrophoblasts and syncytiotrophoblasts, respectively). PSTT is derived from the intermediate trophoblast in the implantation site, whereas ETT is derived from the intermediate trophoblast of the chorion laeve (chorionic-type intermediate trophoblast) [21].

Microscopically, PSTT appears as infiltrating sheets and nests of monomorphic intermediate trophoblasts in the myometrium or endomyometrium, with moderate nuclear pleomorphism and mitotic activity. Chorionic villi are rarely found. On IHC, these tumours stain positive for human placental lactogen (hPL), MUC4, Mel-Cam (CD146) and HLA-G. A majority of tumours are also positive for GATA 3 while hCG can be focally positive [10, 13, 21]. PDL1 expression has also been reported in these tumours. SALL4 immunohistochemical staining may help in differentiating PSTT from choriocarcinoma as the former does not express SALL4 [22]. Pregnancy-associated major basic protein (pMBP) is a marker for intermediate trophoblasts and has been found to stain positively in PSTT [23].

ETT is composed of a uniform population of mononucleate intermediate trophoblasts, with distinct hyalinisation forming nests and solid sheets. Compared to PSTT, ETT shows a nested nodular growth. These tumours express epithelial antigens, alpha inhibin and stain diffusely positive with p63, PLAP and cytokeratin. The hCG and hPL positivity is weak and scattered. Positive immunostaining for p63 differentiates it from PSTT [8, 10, 13].

ETT can be confused with keratinising squamous cell carcinoma due to their epithelioid histology, associated hyaline-like material resembling keratin and the site of involvement (lower uterine segment and cervix) [8, 13]. The two can be differentiated on immunohistochemistry, as SCC does not express alpha inhibin and hPL. On genetic testing, SCC will have only the patient's genetic material, whereas ETT will contain paternally derived genes from the patient's partner as well [5, 10].

Exaggerated placental site reaction (EPSR) and placental site nodule (PSN) are two benign lesions arising from the intermediate trophoblasts [21]. These lesions are usually an incidental finding in pathology specimens after hysterectomy or in uterine curettage tissue. About 14% of atypical placental site nodule (APSN) cases (PSN with atypical features) were found to be associated with malignant

Table 13.1 FIGO staging [25]

Stage I	Tumour confined to the uterus.
Stage II	Tumour extends to other genital structures (ovary, tube, vagina, broad ligaments) by metastasis or direct extension.
Stage III	Pulmonary metastasis with or without pelvic involvement.
Stage IV	All other distant metastasis.

disease—PSTT and ETT, either concurrently or subsequently within months of APSN diagnosis [24]. Hence, the presence of APSN on curettage specimen warrants detailed workup and close follow-up.

13.5 Staging

FIGO staging for GTN (Table 13.1) alone is used to decide treatment. The WHO scoring system, which is used in other GTN patients for risk assessment, is not found to be useful in PSTT and ETT patients [3].

13.6 Prognostic Factors

Due to the limited number of cases of PSTT and ETT, establishing risk factors is difficult.

However, the stage of disease at the time of presentation is the most important prognostic factor for survival [3, 12, 26]. A review of 108 cases reported stage as the most significant prognostic factor and stage IV disease was found to be the most critical risk indicator [1]. Schmid et al. reported a 10-year probability of overall survival of 90% in patients with stage I disease while it drops to 52% for stage II and 49% for stages III/IV disease [2].

Another important prognostic factor is the time interval between diagnosis and the antecedent pregnancy event [1, 2, 9, 26]. A UK clinical series of 62 cases found that time since antecedent pregnancy was the significant prognostic factor for overall and recurrence-free survival [2]. All patients with antecedent interval of >48 months died of disease, even if the disease initially appeared to be localised to the uterus. By contrast, almost all patients (98%) presenting within 4 years survived, even though some had metastatic disease. A review of 34 cases from Charing Cross Hospital reported an antecedent interval of >4 years as a risk factor for death [3]. Another review of 55 cases reported an antecedent interval > 2 years as an adverse prognostic factor [9].

Other poor prognostic variables reported are age more than 35 years, number and site of metastasis, maximum hCG levels >1000 mu/ml, previous full-term pregnancy, deep myometrial invasion, extensive coagulative necrosis, high mitotic count, presence of cells with clear cytoplasm and lymphovascular invasion [2, 9, 26, 27].

13.7 Treatment of PSTT and ETT

13.7.1 Uterine Confined Disease [15, 25]

Recommended treatment for stage I disease includes hysterectomy with lymph nodal assessment and dissection of enlarged pelvic and retroperitoneal lymph nodes. The incidence of lymph node involvement in patients with disease clinically confined to the uterus is about 5–15%; therefore, lymph node biopsy is recommended, especially in large, deeply invasive tumours. Ovarian preservation is recommended unless the patient is postmenopausal or has other indication for oophorectomy. Adjuvant treatment is individualised depending on the histopathological features and interval from antecedent pregnancy (Table 13.2).

Surveillance with clinical examination, imaging and hCG (if elevated initially) are recommended in the absence of the above risk factors.

Adjuvant systemic chemotherapy is recommended for patients with poor prognostic factors, similar to the management of metastatic disease. It is advocated to give combination chemotherapy for 8 weeks (3 cycles) after surgery [15].

Although hysterectomy is the standard treatment, fertility-sparing surgical procedures like wedge resection of the uterus or dilatation and curettage may be considered in carefully selected patients after proper counselling. A small case series of six patients utilised intravenous and intrauterine arterial infusion of chemotherapy following conservative surgery. Shen et al. reported one successful pregnancy and normal delivery with complete remission in all patients at a mean follow-up of 47 months [28]. This should be only considered in young patients who are desirous to preserve fertility and have responded well to conservative surgery and chemotherapy and have no adverse prognostic factors on histopathology. Pfeffer et al. have also reported fertility-sparing partial hysterectomy in PSTT [29]. However, these patients should be carefully counselled as multifocal microscopic disease may be present.

13.7.2 Metastatic/Recurrent Disease [15, 25]

A combination of chemotherapy and surgery is recommended for metastatic disease. These tumours are relatively chemoresistant, and residual masses remaining after chemotherapy may harbour microscopic disease. Surgery has an important role in PSTT/ETT; hence, hysterectomy with excision of metastatic disease

Table 13.2 Indications for adjuvant treatment—poor prognostic factors [25]

1. Interval from index pregnancy ≥2 years
2. Deep myometrial invasion
3. Necrosis
4. Mitotic count >5/10 HPFs

Table 13.3 Chemotherapy regimens for PSTT/ETT [25]

1. EMA/EP	Etoposide, methotrexate, dactinomycin/etoposide, cisplatin
2. EP/EMA	Etoposide, cisplatin/etoposide, methotrexate, dactinomycin
3. TP/TE	Paclitaxel, cisplatin/paclitaxel, etoposide
4. BEP	Bleomycin, etoposide, cisplatin
5. VIP	Etoposide, ifosfamide, cisplatin
6. ICE	Ifosfamide, carboplatin, etoposide

Table 13.4 EMA/EP regimen [25]

EMA/EP—Etoposide, methotrexate, dactinomycin/etoposide, cisplatin (repeat every 2 weeks)
• Etoposide 100 mg/m^2/day IV on days 1 and 2. • Methotrexate 100 mg/m^2 IV push followed by 200 mg/m^2 IV infusion over 12 hours on day 1. • Leucovorin 15 mg PO or IM every 12 hours for 4 doses starting 24 hours after the start of methotrexate. • Dactinomycin 0.5 mg IV push on days 1 and 2.
• Etoposide 100 mg/m^2 IV on day 8. • Cisplatin 75 mg/m^2 IV on day 8.
• Filgrastim 300 mcg SC on days 9–14 of each treatment cycle.

Table 13.5 TP/TE regimen [25]

TP/TE: Paclitaxel, cisplatin/paclitaxel, etoposide (repeat every 2 weeks)
• Paclitaxel 135 mg/m^2 IV infusion on day 1. • Cisplatin 75 mg/m^2 on day 1.
Alternating every 2 weeks with: • Paclitaxel 135 mg/m^2 IV infusion on day 15. • Etoposide 150 mg/m^2 IV on day 15. • Administer pegfilgrastim, 6 mg SC on days 2 and 16.

wherever feasible is recommended. Chemotherapy regimens containing platinum and etoposide like EMA/EP or TP/TE are recommended. Other regimens that can be used in PSTT/ETT are EP/EMA, BEP, VIP or ICE. Myelosuppression is an important side effect associated with these chemotherapy protocols, which may mandate delay and/or dose reduction in subsequent cycles. To overcome neutropenia and avoid delay in the regimes, granulocyte stimulating factor (Filgrastim) is routinely given with each treatment cycle. Chemotherapy is continued for 8 weeks of normal hCG levels. The various chemotherapy regimens recommended for use in PSTT/ETT are listed in Table 13.3. Commonly used regimens with their dosages, namely EMA/EP and TP/TE, are listed in Tables 13.4 and 13.5, respectively.

Other regimens have been tried for chemoresistant and recurrent disease. These include 5-fluorouracil with capecitabine and gemcitabine with or without carboplatin [25]. The role of high-dose chemotherapy (HDC) with peripheral blood stem cell support has also been explored [30]. Targeted biological agents like Pembrolizumab and Nivolumab have also been tried in these patients [25, 31]. However, resistant and recurrent PSTT/ETT can be very difficult to treat and in case of failure of multiple regimens, the best supportive care is what can be offered.

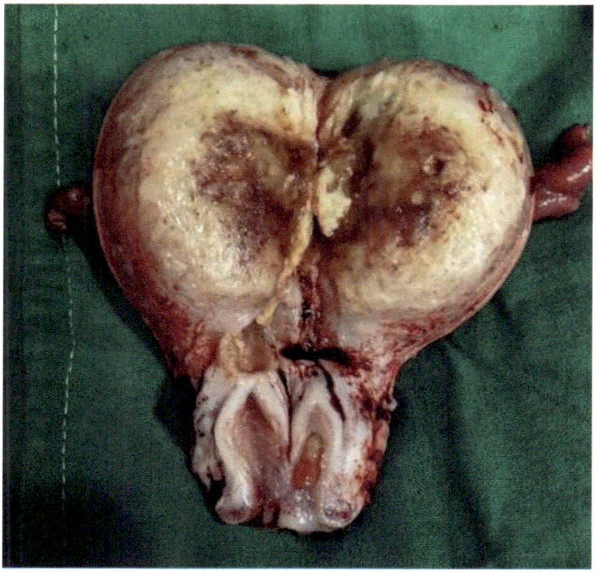

Fig. 13.1 Hysterectomy specimen of a case of PSTT

Of mention here is our own experience with a case of advanced stage PSTT/ETT (unpublished case report, Fig. 13.1). The patient presented 18 months after full-term delivery with gross ascites, mild B/L pleural effusion and endometrial mass invading myometrium. Her hCG at presentation was 163, ascitic fluid was negative for malignancy and endometrial biopsy showed PSTT. The patient had received ten doses of alternate day Methotrexate at an outside hospital before she came to TMH. She underwent a total abdominal hysterectomy with B/L salpingectomy at our centre. The final histopathology report showed PSTT with deep myometrial invasion and areas of necrosis, but mitotic activity was only 1–2/10 HPF and antecedent pregnancy was <2 years; hence, adjuvant treatment was not given. Her hCG values came to normal postsurgery and the patient is disease-free for 19 months.

13.8 Survival

Overall survival has been reported around 90% in patients with stage I disease, 52% for stage II disease and 49% for stage III/IV disease [2]. Worst survival rates are reported for stage IV disease and antecedent interval of more than 4 years [1–3]. The risk of relapse is higher for PSTT and ETT as compared to other GTN and poor outcomes for relapsed disease have been reported, with only 33% of patients achieving remission [2, 32]. The death rates for PSTT/ETT are also higher than other GTN [5].

13.9 Follow-Up and Long-Term Implications

Surveillance is recommended with hCG monitoring and imaging, as hCG alone may not be a reliable marker in these tumours. PET CT can be used for follow-up; it is recommended at the completion of chemotherapy and then every 6–12 months for 2–3 years [25].

Rustin et al. reported an increased risk of developing secondary malignancies in patients receiving combination chemotherapy for GTN [33]. They reported an overall 50% excess of risk in these patients, especially for leukaemia, colon and breast cancers. Leukaemia developed only in patients who received etoposide and other cytotoxic drugs. This warrants long-term monitoring for the treated patients.

13.10 Conclusion

PSTT and ETT are rare forms of GTN with different biological behaviour. They can occur months or years after the index pregnancy event and can follow any type of pregnancy. These tumours grow slowly, remaining confined to the uterus for prolonged periods of time and metastasis usually occurs late in the course of disease. They are chemoresistant and surgery is the mainstay of treatment in both early and advanced stages. The flowchart in Fig. 13.2 lays an outline for the management for PSTT/ETT.

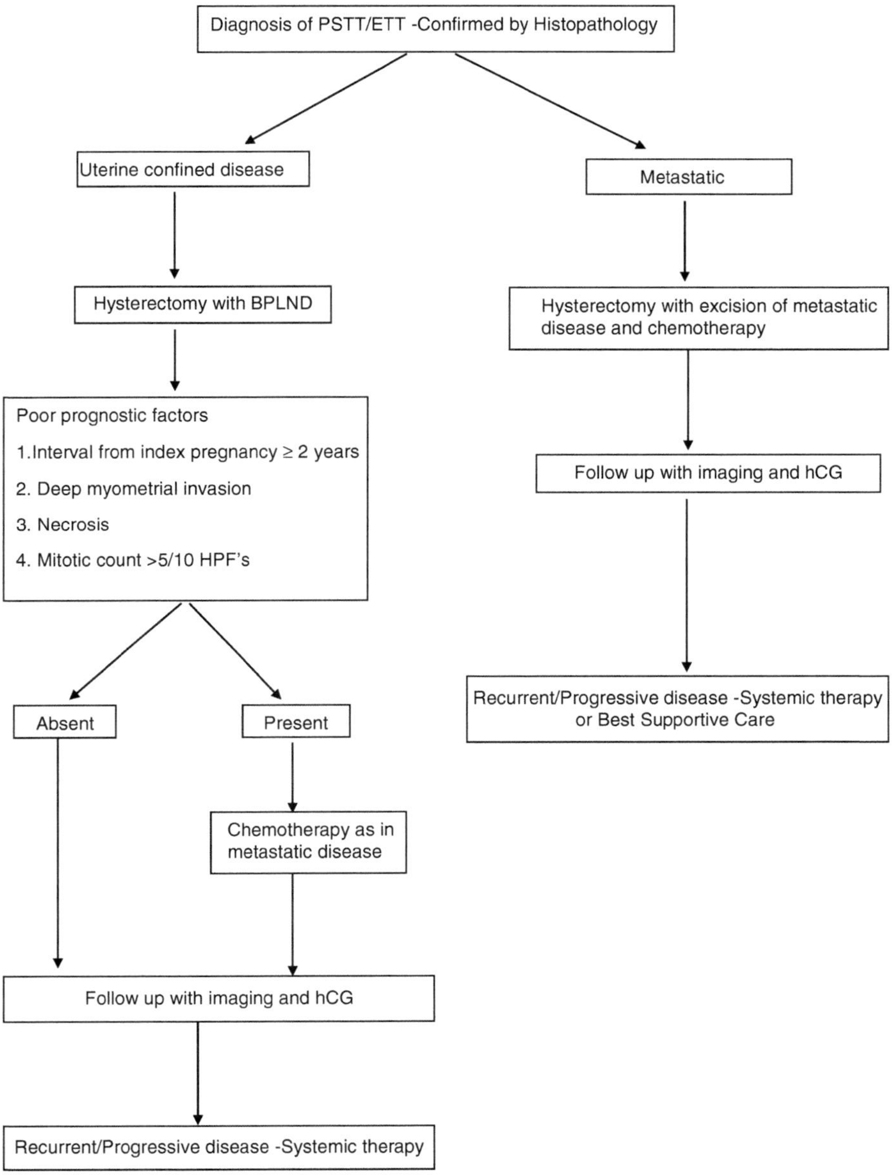

Fig. 13.2 Flowchart for management of PSTT/ETT

References

1. Zhao J, Lv WG, Feng FZ, Wan XR, Liu JH, Yi XF, et al. Placental site trophoblastic tumor: a review of 108 cases and their implications for prognosis and treatment. Gynecol Oncol. 2016;142(1):102–8.
2. Schmid P, Nagai Y, Agarwal R, Hancock B, Savage PM, Sebire NJ, et al. Prognostic markers and long-term outcome of placental-site trophoblastic tumours: a retrospective observational study. Lancet Lond Engl. 2009;374(9683):48–55.
3. Papadopoulos AJ, Foskett M, Seckl MJ, McNeish I, Paradinas FJ, Rees H, et al. Twenty-five years' clinical experience with placental site trophoblastic tumors. J Reprod Med. 2002 Jun;47(6):460–4.
4. Horowitz NS, Goldstein DP, Berkowitz RS. Placental site trophoblastic tumors and epithelioid trophoblastic tumors: biology, natural history, and treatment modalities. Gynecol Oncol. 2017 Jan;144(1):208–14.
5. Hancock BW, Seckl MJ. Placental site and epithelioid trophoblastic tumours. Chapter 20, GTD book. https://www.isstd.org.
6. Kurman RJ, Scully RE, Norris HJ. Trophoblastic pseudotumor of the uterus: an exaggerated form of "syncytial endometritis" simulating a malignant tumor. Cancer. 1976;38(3):1214–26.
7. Scully RE, Young RH. Trophoblastic pseudotumor: a reappraisal. Am J Surg Pathol. 1981;5(1):75.
8. Shih IM, Kurman RJ. Epithelioid trophoblastic tumor: a neoplasm distinct from choriocarcinoma and placental site trophoblastic tumor simulating carcinoma. Am J Surg Pathol. 1998;22(11):1393–403.
9. Baergen RN, Rutgers JL, Young RH, Osann K, Scully RE. Placental site trophoblastic tumor: a study of 55 cases and review of the literature emphasizing factors of prognostic significance. Gynecol Oncol. 2006;100(3):511–20.
10. Sebire NJ, Kaur B, Wells M. Pathology. Chapter 4, GTD book. https://www.isstd.org.
11. Palmer JE, Macdonald M, Wells M, Hancock BW, Tidy JA. Epithelioid trophoblastic tumor: a review of the literature. J Reprod Med. 2008;53(7):465–75.
12. Hyman DM, Bakios L, Gualtiere G, Carr C, Grisham RN, Makker V, et al. Placental site trophoblastic tumor: analysis of presentation, treatment, and outcome. Gynecol Oncol. 2013;129(1):58–62.
13. Shet T, Parage M, Maheshwari A, Nair R, Gupta S, Tongaonkar H, et al. Epithelioid trophoblastic tumor of uterus presenting as an ovarian mass: a diagnostic and therapeutic dilemma. Indian J Pathol Microbiol. 2008 Jun;51(2):242–4.
14. Lan C, Li Y, He J, Liu J. Placental site trophoblastic tumor: lymphatic spread and possible target markers. Gynecol Oncol. 2010 Mar;116(3):430–7.
15. Gestational trophoblastic disease: ESMO clinical practice guidelines | ESMO [Internet]. [cited 2019 Aug 30]. Retrieved from https://www.esmo.org/Guidelines/Gynaecological-Cancers/Gestational-Trophoblastic-Disease
16. Moutte A, Doret M, Hajri T, Peyron N, Chateau F, Massardier J, et al. Placental site and epithelioid trophoblastic tumours: diagnostic pitfalls. Gynecol Oncol. 2013;128(3):568–72.
17. Cole LA, Khanlian SA, Muller CY. Blood test for placental site trophoblastic tumor and non-trophoblastic malignancy for evaluating patients with low positive human chorionic gonadotropin results. J Reprod Med. 2008;53(7):457–64.
18. Zhou Y, Lu H, Yu C, Tian Q, Lu W. Sonographic characteristics of placental site trophoblastic tumor. Ultrasound Obstet Gynecol. 2013;41(6):679–84.
19. Qin J, Ying W, Cheng X, Wu X, Lu B, Liang Y, et al. A well-circumscribed border with peripheral Doppler signal in sonographic image distinguishes epithelioid trophoblastic tumor from other gestational trophoblastic neoplasms. PLoS One. 2014;9(11):e112618.
20. Seckl MJ, Sebire NJ, Berkowitz RS. Gestational trophoblastic disease. Lancet Lond Engl. 2010;376(9742):717–29.

21. Shih IM, Kurman RJ. The pathology of intermediate trophoblastic tumors and tumor-like lesions. Int J Gynecol Pathol. 2001 Jan;20(1):31–47.
22. Stichelbout M, Devisme L, Franquet-Ansart H, Massardier J, Vinatier D, Renaud F, et al. SALL4 expression in gestational trophoblastic tumors: a useful tool to distinguish choriocarcinoma from placental site trophoblastic tumor and epithelioid trophoblastic tumor. Hum Pathol. 2016;54:121–6.
23. Rhoton-Vlasak A, Wagner JM, Rutgers JL, Baergen RN, Young RH, Roche PC, et al. Placental site trophoblastic tumor: human placental lactogen and pregnancy-associated major basic protein as immunohistologic markers. Hum Pathol. 1998;29(3):280–8.
24. Kaur B, Short D, Fisher RA, Savage PM, Seckl MJ, Sebire NJ. Atypical placental site nodule (APSN) and association with malignant gestational trophoblastic disease; a clinicopathologic study of 21 cases. Int J Gynecol Pathol. 2015;34(2):152–8.
25. Gestational Trophoblastic Neoplasia: NCCN guidelines. Available from: https://www.nccn.org/professionals/physician_gls/pdf/gtn.pdf.
26. Frijstein MM, Lok CAR, van Trommel NE, Ten Kate-Booij MJ, LFAG M, van Werkhoven E, et al. Management and prognostic factors of epithelioid trophoblastic tumors: results from the International Society for the Study of trophoblastic diseases database. Gynecol Oncol. 2019;152(2):361–7.
27. Feltmate CM, Genest DR, Wise L, Bernstein MR, Goldstein DP, Berkowitz RS. Placental site trophoblastic tumor: a 17-year experience at the New England trophoblastic disease Center. Gynecol Oncol. 2001 Sep;82(3):415–9.
28. Shen X, Xiang Y, Guo L, Feng F, Wan X, Xiao Y, et al. Fertility-preserving treatment in young patients with placental site trophoblastic tumors. Int J Gynecol Cancer. 2012;22(5):869–74.
29. Pfeffer PE, Sebire N, Lindsay I, McIndoe A, Lim A, Seckl MJ. Fertility-sparing partial hysterectomy for placental-site trophoblastic tumour. Lancet Oncol. 2007 Aug;8(8):744–6.
30. Frijstein MM, Lok CAR, Short D, Singh K, Fisher RA, Hancock BW, et al. The results of treatment with high-dose chemotherapy and peripheral blood stem cell support for gestational trophoblastic neoplasia. Eur J Cancer. 2019 Mar;109:162–71.
31. Ghorani E, Kaur B, Fisher RA, Short D, Joneborg U, Carlson JW, et al. Pembrolizumab is effective for drug-resistant gestational trophoblastic neoplasia. Lancet Lond Engl. 2017;390(10110):2343–5.
32. Zhang X, Lü W, Lü B. Epithelioid trophoblastic tumor: an outcome-based literature review of 78 reported cases. Int J Gynecol Cancer. 2013;23(7):1334–8.
33. Rustin GJ, Newlands ES, Lutz JM, Holden L, Bagshawe KD, Hiscox JG, et al. Combination but not single-agent methotrexate chemotherapy for gestational trophoblastic tumors increases the incidence of second tumors. J Clin Oncol. 1996 Oct;14(10):2769–73.

Critical Situations in Gestational Trophoblastic Diseases

14

Bhagyalaxmi Nayak and Sweta Singh

14.1 Introduction

Gestational trophoblastic diseases (GTD) are a group of heterogenous disease that arise from trophoblast; and range from premalignant conditions like partial and complete hydatidiform moles to malignant lesions like invasive hydatidiform moles, choriocarcinoma and the rarer placental site trophoblastic and epithelioid tumours [1–7]. The malignant forms of the disease that will need chemotherapy are collectively called gestational trophoblastic neoplasms (GTN) [1].

The incidence of GTD is higher in Asian (1 in 500) and African (1 in 1000) than European or American (1 in 1500) population [3, 4, 7]. The incidence of molar pregnancy in India is 1 in 400 pregnancies [8]. About 80% of GTDs are hydatidiform moles. Risk factors for the development of hydatidiform moles include extremes of age, ethnicity, history of spontaneous miscarriage and dietary deficiencies [9]. Women between 21 and 35 years of age have a lower incidence than women younger than 21 years or older than 35 years [10]. The etiopathology, diagnosis, presentation and management of GTDs have been described previously. This chapter will outline the critical situations encountered with GTDs.

14.2 Critical Events

GTDs entail a variety of presentations secondary to their endocrine, secretory, angiogenic and other properties. Presentations may sometimes be extremely perplexing and not fit into any clinical situation. Presentation may be sometimes so

B. Nayak (✉)
Associate Professor, Department of Gynaecologic Oncology, Regional Cancer Center, Cuttack, India

S. Singh
Department of Obstetrics and Gynaecology, AIIMS Bhubaneswar, Bhubaneswar, India

B. Nayak, U. Singh (eds.), *Gestational Trophoblastic Disease*,
https://doi.org/10.1007/978-981-33-4878-3_14

acute that GTD is occasionally diagnosed for the first time in ICU. The presentation is often acute or subacute and clinicians need to keep a high risk of suspicion of GTDs in all women in the reproductive age group [11].

14.2.1 Haemorrhage

Excessive vaginal bleeding is known to occur with GTDs [11]. This may be due to the production of high levels of angiogenic growth factors which remodel the uterine vasculature and lead to the formation of arteriovenous malformation. Although more commonly seen in choriocarcinoma, abnormal uterine bleeding may be seen in complete hydatidiform mole and placental-site trophoblastic disease [11]. Due to the chance of significant bleeding during procedures like suction evacuation of hydatidiform mole, RCOG guidelines (2010) advocate the presence of a senior surgeon (Fig. 14.1) [12]. Blood should also be kept cross-matched in the event of sudden post-procedure haemorrhage. Bleeding and shock does sometimes occur remote from the procedure. Hence proper counselling for a strict followup and appraisal of complications that could ensue will go a long way in reducing the preventable morbidity and mortality.

The use of oxytocics before the evacuation of molar pregnancy is not recommended because of the theoretical concern of the trophoblastic material embolising through the uterine venous plexus into the systemic veins [12]. However, to control life-threatening bleeding, infusions of oxytocics may be required. Similarly, preparation of the cervix with prostaglandins and use of sharp curettage is also not recommended [13]. Apart from major bleeding during the evacuation of molar pregnancy,

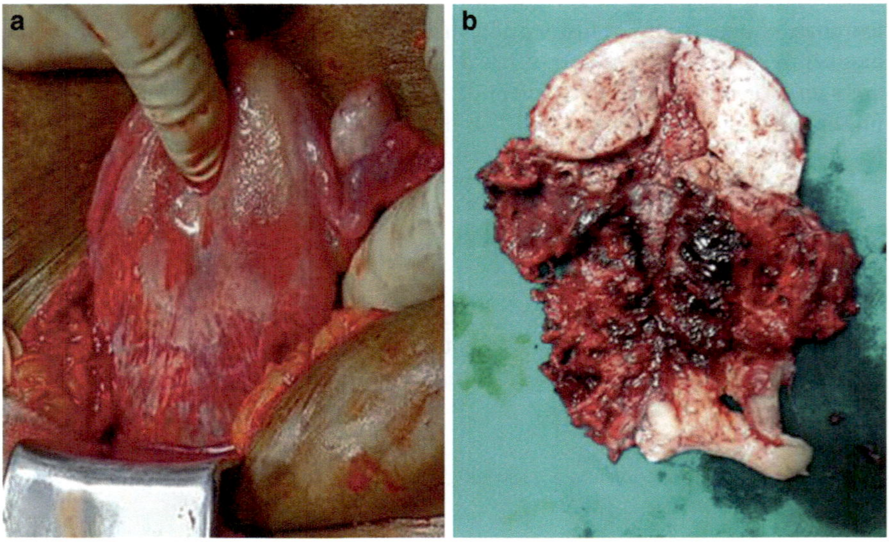

Fig. 14.1 Invasive mole—Patient had torrential haemorrhage during attempted suction and evacuation. (**a**) Emergency laparotomy and (**b**) cut open gross specimen showing invasive mole

acute cardiopulmonary distress and adult respiratory distress syndrome have also been reported after suction evacuation in 27% of cases.

Haemorrhage may not be only confined to vaginal bleeding. Excessive haemorrhage has also been reported in the gastrointestinal tract and patients may present with excessive haematemesis and melena or lower gastrointestinal tract bleeding [14, 15]. Unexplained anaemia is often seen in these patients and may or may not be associated with masses in the small bowel or colon [16]. Rarer manifestations include recurrent epistaxis along with abnormal vaginal and rectal bleeding [11]. Bleeding leading to a painful eye with decreased visual acuity has also been reported [11]. Torrential bleeding may happen from suburetrhral nodule (Fig. 14.2). Stitches may be difficult to fix. Styptics , local and systemic, with packing may be helpful at times. Hence biopsy from such nodules is not only unnecassary but may be lethal at times.

14.2.2 Perforation and Spontaneous Uterine Rupture

There are case reports of spontaneous uterine perforation in patients with choriocarcinoma [17, 18]. The possible mechanisms are invasion of blood vessels by the trophoblastic cells leading to uterine infarction at multiple sites due to thrombosis, aneurysm formation and tumoral bleeding [11]. Other possible causes of uterine rupture are invasion of the uterine endometrium and myometrium by tumour cells or tumour necrosis due to chemotherapy [11]. Such patients may present with signs and symptoms of acute abdomen and emergency hysterectomy may have to be performed. Massive hemoperitoneum occurring days after suction and evacuation procedure may occur when the invasive component of the disease has been missed or may accrue after the procedure (Fig. 14.3). Hence, thorough counselling of patients for strict follow-up is the onus of the consultant. Treatment is always surgical. Segmental resection is the treatment of choice. The patient is often hemodynamically unstable and hence needs utmost attention.

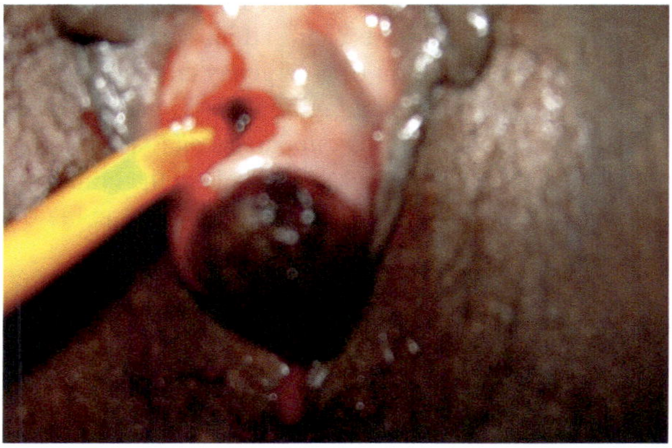

Fig. 14.2 Vaginal nodule in GTD

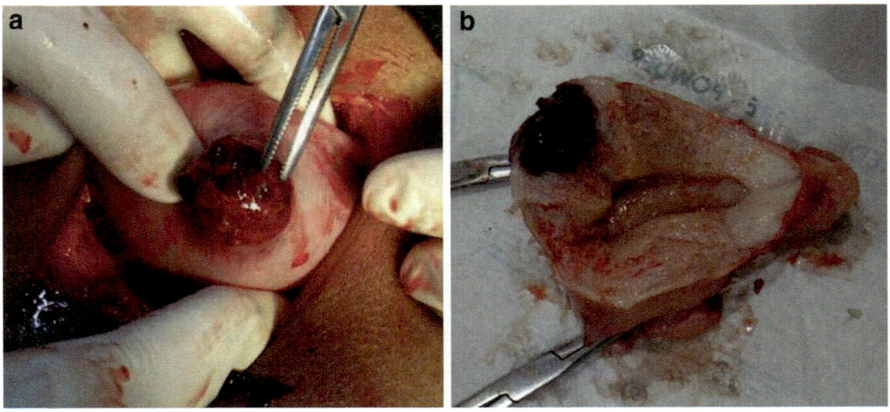

Fig. 14.3 Woman presented in emergency after 1 month of molar evacuation with massive hemoperitoneum where laparotomy with hysterectomy was performed. (**a**) Fundal perforation is seen and (**b**) cut section of specimen showing the perforation

14.2.3 Systemic Signs of Tumour Metastasis

The lung parenchyma is the most common site of metastasis in patients with choriocarcinoma and patients may present with signs and symptoms of acute respiratory failure like dyspnoea, acute chest pain with or without haemoptysis [19] and sudden onset of pulmonary hypertension due to pulmonary embolism (Fig. 14.4) [20]. In fact, the differential diagnosis of choriocarcinoma should be kept in mind in a young woman presenting with sudden onset of pulmonary hypertension due to pulmonary embolism without any other antecedent risk factors [11]. Women may land up in pulmonary medicine department leading to delay in treatment and detorioration, which is sometimes acute and sudden. Hence a element of suspicion in women of reproductive age group is worth a life.

Central nervous system involvement occurs in 10% of patients with choriocarcinoma and has varied manifestations [11]. Tumour metastasis to the central nervous system is also common which manifests as raised intracranial pressures and seizures [11]. Surgical intervention in the form of emergency craniotomy to release intracranial pressure has been done with encouraging results. Sudden onset of stroke-like symptoms have also been reported with hemiparesis and facial palsy due to multiple intracerebral haemorrhages from aneurysmal vessels in the brain [21]. Though challenging, treatment of seemingly hopeless cases does benefit in majority of cases.

14.2.4 Acute Abdomen

Acute abdomen has been reported in patients with GTDs due to rupture and haemorrhage, intussusception and extrauterine sites of implantation mimicking ruptured

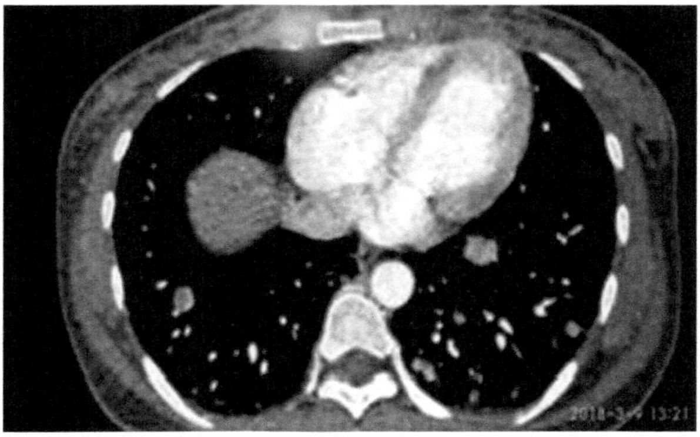

Fig. 14.4 CECT thorax showing multiple lung metastases in a patient of GTN presenting with haemoptysis where chest X-ray was inconclusive

ectopic pregnancy [11, 22]. Massive intraperitoneal haemorrhage has also been reported but may be due to variable aetiology like ruptured liver or spleen or a ruptured blood vessel [11]. Involvement of the kidney causes symptoms and signs of acute flank pain with hematuria and renovascular hypertension [23]. In fact, on many occasions, the abdomen has been opened suspecting ruptured ectopic or intestinal perforation and has been later found to be GTD [11]. GTD of fallopian tubes may present exactly like ruptured ectopic and proved only by a postoperative histopathologic study of the removed appendage.

14.2.5 Thyrotoxicosis

The similar structure of the human chorionic gonadotrophin (hCG) and thyroid-stimulating hormone causes hCG to exert a thyrotrophic action and signs and symptoms of thyrotoxicosis such as hypertension, tachycardia, atrial fibrillation and congestive cardiac failure has been reported in these patients (Fig. 14.5) [24]. So, the differential diagnosis of GTDs should always be kept in mind in a woman after any pregnancy event presenting with signs and symptoms of thyrotoxicosis and both serum hCG as well as thyroid hormone assay should be performed [11].

14.2.6 Acute Vascular Events

Due to the presence of a hypercoagulable state, venous and arterial thromboembolism may occur [25]. Activation of platelets and factors XII and X due to tumour cell–macrophage interaction causes the release of cytokines like TNF-alpha and interleukins leading to endothelial damage. Other risk factors may be the toxicity of chemotherapeutic agents [11].

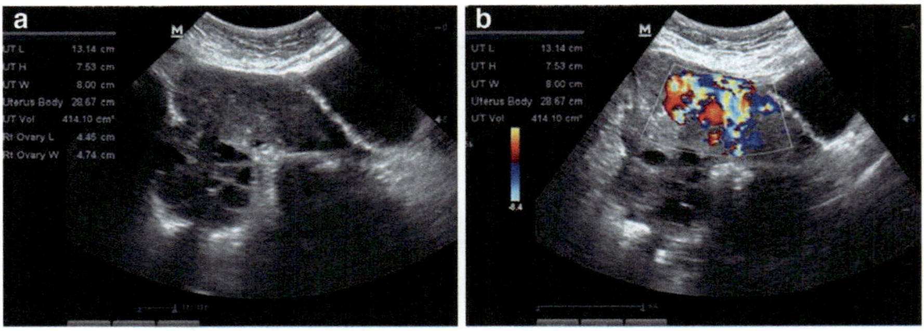

Fig. 14.5 Case of GTN which presented with features of thyrotoxicosis. (**a**) Grey scale 2D ultrasonography showing uterus with theca-lutein cyst of ovary and (**b**) colour Doppler image showing increased vascularity inside the uterus

14.2.7 Sepsis

Clostridium perfringens induced sepsis has been reported in a case of invasive molar pregnancy. The necrotic tumour tissue creates hypoxic and ischaemic conditions that allow the proliferation of this anaerobic Gram-positive bacillus leading to the formation of gas gangrene [26]. In this particular case, the sepsis is resolved after hysterectomy leading to removal of the septic foci [26]. Similarly, previous reports exist of association of clostridium infections in patients with choriocarcinoma [27].

14.2.8 Ovarian Hyperstimulation Syndrome

This condition is typically seen in patients following ovulation induction and consists of enlarged ovaries, with multiple follicular cysts and acute fluid shifts from intravascular space to the extracellular space, causing haemoconcentration, oedema, electrolyte disturbances and massive pleural effusion, ascites and pericardial effusions in severe cases leading to acute thromboembolic events and even death. Although sometimes seen in twin pregnancy, ovarian hyperstimulation syndrome has been reported 3 days after molar pregnancy evacuation [28]. It is likely that the high levels of hCG cause bilateral ovarian stimulation and enlargement. Young women presenting with ascites and enlarged ovaries and raised B HCG may be mistaken for germ cell tumour of ovaries and careful decision needs to be taken along with a history of recent termination of pregnancy.

14.2.9 Chemotherapy

Occasionally very high-risk cases with large tumour burden may present with an acute serious illness due to tumour lysis and haemorrhage. Though seemingly hopeless, careful management of these cases will help them survive as they are potentially curable. Alternatively, low-dose Etoposide 100 mg/m^2 and cisplatin 20 mg/m^2 (EP) induction chemotherapy for patients with high-volume disease is a better and safer option. Ensuring adequate hydration, commencing therapy with allopurinol or rasburicase and special attention to electrolyte balance and renal function has reduced the rates of early deaths [29]. Fatal pulmonary haemorrhage may occur due to positive pressure ventilation as the vessels are very friable; hence, low pressure is recommended. Tumour lysis may sometimes lead to multiorgan failure and death. Life-threatening myelosuppression is sometimes a crisis to manage vigourously.

14.2.10 Critical Situations During Surgery

There is a chance of embolisation of the trophoblastic tissue; hence, minimal manipulation and prophylactic or perioperative CT is proposed by some to be another method to prevent embolisation. Patients are usually anaemic and hemodynamically unstable and need added attention and precaution. Extensive vascular supply and the friable nature of the uterus may lead to extensive intra-op blood loss that has to be handled properly and fast. Sometimes, unrecognised extrauterine disease may pose a challenge. DIC, though rare, should be kept in mind. Hence, it is always advisable to handle surgery in GTD by an experienced surgical team along with an adequate blood transfusion facility and ICU backup.

14.2.11 Unstable Patients

An extensive metastatic burden and hCG levels of over 500,000 IU/L behave unpredictably. An initial treatment with MTX infusion/leucovorin rescue or Etoposide 100 mg/m^2 ± cisplatin 50–75 mg/m^2 is sometimes given to avoid catastrophic haemorrhage from high-risk sites of metastases. EMA/CO is initiated as soon as the condition improves.

14.2.12 Adnexal Torsion and Theca Leutin Cyst Rupture

Present with acute abdomen and need immediate treatment.

14.2.13 Thyroid Crisis

High levels of HCG are typically required for the development of clinical hyperthyroidism. Iodinated substances can trigger a crisis (**Jod Basedow phenomenon).** Rarely the thyroid stimulation can have potentially life-threatening consequences. Carbimazole and β-blockers for symptom relief appear to be effective. Thyroid function normalises rapidly with treatment of the underlying GTD and the consequent fall in HCG levels [30].

14.3 Conclusion

GTDs constitute a clinical conundrum and often the first presentation to the hospital is because of an acute or subacute crisis. Clinicians will likely encounter such women in their practice and therefore need to be aware of the varied critical events that may manifest in these women. Often, the diagnosis may not be readily apparent as the heterogeneity of the disease leads to signs and symptoms that are present in other organs. Therefore, a high index of suspicion of GTDs should be kept in mind while attending to women in the reproductive age group presenting with an acute or subacute crisis. Overall, definitive care for GTN is the purview of the gynaecologist but the emergency physicians should be aware of the risks and be able to recognise the patient with this potentially lethal but curable disease.

References

1. Seckl MJ. Gestational trophoblastic disease: clinical presentation and treatment. Diagn Histopathol. 2018;25(2):77–85.
2. Ngan HY, Seckl MJ, Berkowitz RS, et al. Update on the diagnosis and management of gestational trophoblastic disease. Int J Gynaecol Obstet. 2015;131(suppl 2):S123–6.
3. Steigrad SJ. Epidemiologyofgestationaltrophoblasticdiseases. Best Pract Res Clin Obstet Gynaecol. 2003;17(6):837–47.
4. Altieri A, Franceschi S, Ferlay J, Smith J, La Vecchia C. Epidemiology and aetiology of gestational trophoblastic diseases. Lancet Oncol. 2003;4(11):670–8.
5. Martin BH, Kim JH. Changes in gestational trophoblastic tumors over four decades: a Korean experience. J Reprod Med. 1998;43(1):60–8.
6. Seckl MJ, Sebire NJ, Berkowitz RS. Gestationaltrophoblastic disease. Lancet. 2010;376(9742):717–29.
7. Lurain JR. Gestationaltrophoblasticdisease. I. Epidemiology, pathology, clinical presentation and diagnosis of gestational trophoblastic disease, and management of hydatidiform mole. Am J Obstet Gynecol. 2010;203(6):531–9.
8. Dutta DC. Haemorrhage in early pregnancy. In: Konan H, editor. Textbook of obstetrics. 6th ed. Kolkata: New Central Book Agency; 2004. p. 159–202.
9. Nadhan R, Vaman JV, Nirmala C, et al. Insights into dovetailing GTD and cancers. Crit Rev Oncol Hematol. 2017;114:77–90.
10. Newlands ES, Paradinas FJ, Fisher RA. Recent advances in gestational trophoblastic disease. Hematol Oncol Clin North Am. 1999;13(1):225–44.
11. Mangla M, Singla D, Kaur H, Sharma S. Unusual clinical presentations of choriocarcinoma: a systematic review of case reports. Taiwan J Obstet Gynecol. 2017;56:1–8.
12. The management of gestational trophoblastic diseases. Green-top guidelines. Royal College of Obstetricians and Gynaecologists. 2010. p. 1–12.
13. Stone M, Bagshawe KD. An analysis of the influences of maternal age, gestational age, contraceptive method, and the mode of primary treatment of patients with hydatidiform moles on the incidence of subsequent chemotherapy. Br J Obstet Gynaecol. 1979;86(10):782–92.
14. Villet WT, Du Toit DF, Conroy C. Unusual presentation of choriocarcinoma. A case report. S Afr Med J. 1979;55:96e8.
15. Suski E, Pavlides C, Matsumoto T. Massive lower gastrointestinal bleeding: unusual presentation of metastatic choriocarcinoma. Int Surg. 1979;64:53e5.
16. Chaturvedi M, Vaideeswar P, Pandit A. Metastatic Choriocarcinoma: an unusual cause of severe anemia. J Postgrad Med. 2005;51:230e1.

17. Xie C, Zheng L, Li Z, Zhao X. Spontaneous uterine perforation of choriocarcinoma with negative beta-human chorionic gonadotropin after chemotherapy. Med Princ Pract. 2011;20:570e3.
18. Okamoto T, Nomura S, Nakanishi T, Yamada S, Tomoda Y. A case of uterine choriocarcinoma with spontaneous rupture twenty-three years following theantecedent pregnancy. J Obstet Gynaecol Res. 1997;23:189e95.
19. Berkowitz RS, Goldstein DP. Gestational trophoblastic disease. In: Berek J, editor. Berek& Novak's gynecology. Philadelphia: Lippincott Williams & Wilkins; 2007. p. 1581e603.
20. Gangadharan VP, Chitrathara K, Sivaramakrishnan R, Satishkumar K, Nair MK. Pulmonary hypertension: a rare presentation of choriocarcinoma. Acta Oncol. 1993;32:461e2.
21. Daniel CN, Ango IG, Nwobodo EI. Choriocarcinoma with cerebral metastasis presenting as a stroke like lesion. Sahel Med J. 2015;18:16e9.
22. Mittal S, Aird I, Haugk B. Gestational choriocarcinoma in liver mimicking ruptured ectopic pregnancy. J Obstet Gynaecol. 2012;32:499.
23. Usta TA, Karacan T, Ozyurek E, Naki MM, Omeroglu SN, Demirkiran F. Primary renal artery choriocarcinoma causing secondary renovascular hypertension. Int J Surg Case Rep. 2014;5:1197e9.
24. O'Reilly S, Lyons DJ, Harrison M, Gaffney E, Cullen M, Clancy L. Thyrotoxicosis induced by choriocarcinoma a report of two cases. Ir Med J. 1993;86:124e7.
25. Cyriac S, Sagar TG, Mahajan V. Choriocarcinoma with arterial and venous thrombosis. Neurol India. 2009;57:505e7.
26. Singh S, Angra K, Bonnie D, Shokrani B. Complications of invasive molar pregnancy with clostridium perfringes sepsis. Case Rep Obstet Gynaecol. 2014:Article ID 282141.
27. Chern-Horng L, Hsieh SY. Clostridium septicum infection presenting as liver abscess in a case of choriocarcinoma with liver metastasis. J Gastroenterol Hepatol. 1999;14(12):1227–9.
28. Arora R, Merhi ZO, Khulpateea N, et al. Ovarian hyperstimulation syndrome after a molar pregnancy evacuation. Fertil Steril. 2008;90(4):1197.e5–7.
29. Agarwal R, et al. Management and survival of patients with FIGO high-risk gestational trophoblastic neoplasia: the U.K. experience, 1995–2010. J Reprod Med. 2014;59(12):7–12.
30. Walkington L, et al. Hyperthyroidism and human chorionic gonadotropin production in gestational trophoblastic disease. Br J Cancer. 2011;104:1665–9.

Recurrent Molar Pregnancy 15

Sabera Khatun

Molar pregnancy is a gestational trophoblastic disorder as a result of abnormal fertilisation and gametogenesis, characterised by hydropic swelling of the placental villi, hyperplasia of villous trophoblast and absent, or abnormal, faetal development. It is potentially a malignant pregnancy condition, broadly grouped under gestational trophoblastic disease (GTD). The commonest molar pregnancy is complete hydatidiform mole (CHM) and the next common is partial hydatidiform mole (PHM). The malignant form of GTD is otherwise called gestational trophoblastic neoplasia (GTN) which encompasses: Invasive mole (IM), Choriocarcinoma (CCA), Placental site trophoblastic tumour (PSTT) and Epitheloid trophoblastic tumour (ETT). More than 80% of molar pregnancies are cured with usual suction and evacuation with regular follow-up with clinical and β-hCG estimation. About 15–20% of CHM and 3–5% of PHM will require chemotherapy depending upon the WHO score for GTN with normal pregnancy outcome thereafter. However, it is typical that once molar pregnancy, there is a high risk of molar events in subsequent pregnancy. By definition, recurrent hydatidiform mole is characterised by the occurrences of at least two abnormal pregnancies that have resulted in hydatidiform mole.

15.1 Recurrence Rate in Complete and Partial Molar Pregnancy

The incidence of molar pregnancy varies widely from country to country, even from one part of the same country to other parts. It is estimated that 1 in 1000 pregnancies in most parts of the world [1] and 2 in 1000 pregnancies in the Asian population do have molar pregnancy events [2]. Savage et al. observed recurrent HM in 1 in 68 in a 10 years survey of over 5000 post-molar pregnancies and concluded that there is

S. Khatun (✉)
Gynecological Oncology Department, Bangabandhu Sheikh Mujib Medical University, Dhaka, Bangladesh

B. Nayak, U. Singh (eds.), *Gestational Trophoblastic Disease*,
https://doi.org/10.1007/978-981-33-4878-3_15

almost tenfold (incidence of molar pregnancy in the UK is 1 in 600 pregnancies) increased chance of repeat mole in subsequent pregnancies following a molar event [3]. Sebire et al. in 2003 also had a similar opinion. They observed an increase of about 1–2% incidence of repeat mole and an increase up to 23% after two consecutive molar pregnancies [4].

Retrospective observation of 16,523 women with first molar pregnancy at Charing Cross Hospital, UK, revealed incidence of second molar pregnancy to be 1% and more common with CHM than PHM (0.91% vs. 0.28%, respectively). The risk of further molar event after one or more non-molar intervening pregnancy was also more in CHM than in PHM (0.65% vs. 0.37%). More than 80% of recurrent moles were of the same histological type as of previous pregnancy. In a study, of 8553 women with histological PHM, only 11 (0.13%) had CHM while of the 7037 with CHM, 21 (0.3%) experienced a subsequent PHM in the same patients in their reproductive life [5]. Vegas et al. observed that 50% of complete and 30% of partial moles are at an increased risk of second HM [6]. Amongst the women having second molar pregnancy, 13% were found to have subsequent third molar pregnancy and most of them had previous two pregnancies with CHM and this rarely did happen with PHM. It was also observed that recurrence of third molar does occur within the first 1–2 years of second molar event, regardless of whether a CHM or PHM [5].

15.2 Familial Recurrent Hydatidiform Mole

It is now recognised that women with recurrent molar pregnancies do have a number of patients included under "the familial recurrent hydatidiform mole (FRHM)". This is a rare autosomal recessive condition, where the woman has an inherited predisposition to have recurrent molar pregnancy, most of which are CHM [7]. Two mutant genes, NLRP7 and KHDC 3 L have been recognised to be responsible for 75 and 5% of cases of FRHM, respectively. Genotyping of the complete mole (CM) can be of value for the identification of the women affected by familial recurrent hydatidiform mole. It is well known that CHM is androgenic (AnCHM), while those affected with FRHM are diploid but biparental in origin (BiCHM) [7].

15.2.1 Incidence

Familial recurrent HM is considered an exceedingly rare condition. In medical literature, only 21 families have been reported to date. According to the report of Charing Cross Hospital, UK, the risk of a third HM is mostly associated with CHM, while 1 in 640 women with third recurrence had FRHM. This condition accounted for most, though not all cases of three or more CHM. It is usually recommended to have a genetic evaluation of molar tissue in women with three or more recurrent molar events, to diagnose FRHM, and fertility counselling can be offered [5].

15.2.2 Diagnosis

Recurrent molar pregnancy can be diagnosed by a thorough evaluation of previous pregnancy losses. Among previous pregnancy losses, molar pregnancy is most important as the outcome of this may be life-threatening and it may be recurrent and may recur in families. In this regard, evaluation of confirmatory evidence of previous molar pregnancies like ultrasonography report, serum β-hCG report, surgical note of molar pregnancy, histopathological report, immune-histochemistry report and finally genotyping report if available are very informative. Every gynaecologist or gynaecological oncologist should be careful about keeping all the records and should counsel the patients and her attendants about the importance of keeping all these records. Recurrent second HM can easily be diagnosed by evaluation of the above records.

15.3 Development of Gestational Trophoblastic Neoplasia (GTN)

After the second mole, the incidence of recurrent molar pregnancy increases to between 10 and 23% [4]. It is associated with an increasing risk of development of GTN. The risk of development to GTN is similar both in AnCHM and BiCHM and is 22% after first molar pregnancy, increases to 50% after the second molar event [8]. Management of such a situation does not differ from GTN developing from molar pregnancy.

15.4 Fertility Issue

Though there is a moderate increased risk of second and third molar event after HM, the pregnancy outcome after one or two molar event does not differ, and so also after chemotherapy when given for GTN. It is observed that most patients with two repeat CHM do have Aan CHM and can have normal pregnancy outcome. Women with FRHM usually do have BiCHM and do have little chance of successful pregnancy [4]. However, as suggested earlier, genetic typing of molar tissue should be advised in cases of three or more repeat molar events to differentiate between CHM and FRHM. If detected to have AnCHM, IVF (ICSI) and preimplantation genetic diagnosis (PGD) can reduce recurrence of CHM and successful pregnancy outcome [9, 10]. Women with FRHM need to be treated by IVF with ovum donation to achieve normal pregnancy [10, 11].

15.4.1 A Case Report

A 40-year-old woman reported to me on 29.9.2018 with the complain of amenorrhea for 2 months. She came from a district town of Dhaka division with a report of transabdominal ultrasonography done on 23.9.18, repeated on 26.9.18. Both reports showed molar pregnancies. Her β-hCG done on 23.9.18 was 225,000 mIU/ml. She had a X-ray Chest report which was normal. Her X-ray Chest, CBC, fasting and 2 h after breakfast blood sugar level, serum electrolytes, SGPT, creatinine level, albumin, all were within normal limit. Her cardiac status was normal.

As a mandatory test for evaluation of thyroid status, she had serum TSH and FT4 level measurement on 3.10.18. Her TSH level was 0.02 nmol/L (N-0.55–4.78 nmol/L) and FT4 level was 359.1 pmol/L (N-58.1–140.6 nmol/L).

Regarding her obstetric history, she is married for 20 years but no normal pregnancy. Unfortunately, she became pregnant four times. Each time it was a molar pregnancy and each time she had suction evacuation for molar pregnancy. This was her fifth pregnancy and it was also molar pregnancy. Her first molar pregnancy was in 2005, second in 2006, third in 2007, fourth in 2014 and this was her fifth pregnancy in 2018.

She consulted with me after her fourth pregnancy to know whether she should be pregnant or not and whether her fifth pregnancy will be molar or not. There was no scope for genotyping, as molar tissue was not available at that time. So, she was advised to take a chance. Now, she came with her fifth molar pregnancy and she does not intend to preserve her uterus. So, the decision was taken to do a total abdominal hysterectomy for her. Her hyperthyroidism was managed conservatively by β blocker agent. She underwent TAH with left-sided salpingo-ophorectomy with right salpingectomy with preservation of right ovary on 11.10.18. On the cut section, the endometrial cavity was found distorted by vesicular grape-like structures. The total volume of the vesicular structure was 100 cc. The size of the biggest vesicle was 0.5 cm.

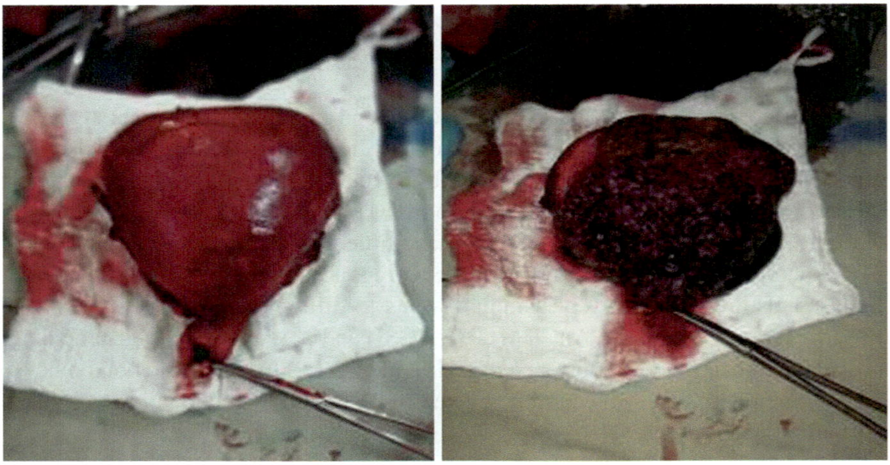

Histopathological report showed complete hydatidiform mole. Serum β-hCG 13.10.18, 48 hours after hysterectomy sharply fell down to 163,541.70 mIU/ml. She was advised to do weekly β-hCG but was reluctant to do so; ultimately she had serum β-hCG on 31.10.18 and it was 267.90 mIU/ml. Her thyroid status become normal and on 16.10.18 serum FT4, FT3 and TSH levels were 27.93 pmol/L, 8.10 p.mol/l and 0.01 mIU/L, respectively. On 7.10.18 it was 19.86, 2.14 and 0.01.

She needs β-hCG done weekly up to three normal levels, then monthly β-hCG done up to 6 months.

15.5 Conclusion

Recurrence of molar pregnancy is a major concern. The recurrence chance of a molar pregnancy to subsequent molar pregnancy is about 1.5–2%, increased to 23% after two or more molar events. Though repeat molar pregnancy does have more chance of development to GTN, treatment and result of treatment do not differ. For better pregnancy outcome, genotyping is recommended in cases of three or more repeat molar events, and ICSI and PGD are employed in androgenic CHM and IVF with ovum donation in biparental CHM may prevent further recurrence and a desirable pregnancy outcome.

References

1. Hancock BW, Seckl MJ, Berkowitz RS. Gestational trophoblastic disease. 4th ed. ISSTD website; 2015. Retrieved from http://test.registraid.com/gtd-book.html. Accessed May 2, 2018.
2. Ngan HY, Seckl MJ, Berkowitz RS, Xiang Y, Golfier F, Sekharan PK, et al. Update on the diagnosis and management of gestational trophoblastic disease. Int J Gynaecol Obstet. 2015;131(Suppl 2):S123–6.
3. Savage PM, Sita-Lumsden A, Dickson S, Iyer R, Everard J, Coleman R, Fisher RA, Short D, Casalboni S, Catalano K, et al. The relationship of maternal age to molar pregnancy incidence, risks for chemotherapy and subsequent pregnancy outcome. J Obstet Gynaecol. 2013;33:406–11.
4. Sebire NJ, Fisher RA, Foskett M, Rees H, Seckl MJ, Newlands ES. Risk of recurrent hydatidiform mole and subsequent pregnancy outcome following complete or partial hydatidiform molar pregnancy. BJOG: An Int J Obstet Gynaecol. 2003;110:22–6.
5. Eagles N, Sebire NJ, Short D, Savage PM, Seck MJ, Fisher RA. Risk of recurrent molar pregnancies following complete and partial hydatidiform moles. Hum Reprod. 2015;30(9):2055–63.
6. Vargas R, Barroilhet LM, Esselen K, Diver E, Bernstein M, Goldstein DP, Berkowitz RS. Subsequent pregnancy outcomes after complete and partial molar pregnancy, recurrent molar pregnancy, and gestational trophoblastic neoplasia: an update from the New England trophoblastic disease Center. J Reprod Med. 2014;59:188–94.
7. Fisher RA, Hodges MD, Newlands ES. Familial recurrent hydatidiform mole: a review. J Reprod Med. 2004;49:595–601.
8. Berkowitz RS, IM SS, Bernstein MR, Goldstein DP. Gestational trophoblastic disease—subsequent pregnancy outcome, including repeat pregnancy. J Reprod Med. 1998;43:81–6.
9. Ogilvie CM, Renwick PJ, Khalaf Y, Braude PR. First use of preimplantation genotyping in prevention of recurrent diandric complete hydatidiform mole. Reprod Biomed Online. 2009;19:224–7.
10. Hafezi M, Chekini Z, Zamanian M. Which one is more prominent in recurrent hydatidiform mole, ovum or sperm? Int J Fertil Steril. 2020;14(2):154–8.
11. Fisher RA, Lavery SA, Carby A, Abu-Hayyeh S, Swingler R, Sebire NJ, Seckl MJ. What a difference an egg makes. Lancet. 2011;378:1974.

16 Fertility Preservation in Gestational Trophoblastic Neoplasia (GTN)

U. D. Bafna

Gestational trophoblastic neoplasia (GTN) consisting of Invasive mole, choriocarcinoma and Placental site trophoblastic tumour (PSTT) have generally good prognosis. They usually follow molar pregnancy but sometimes could occur after an abortion or a term pregnancy. Since these patients are usually young, in reproductive age group and potentially curable fertility preservation should always be the choice of treatment.

The diagnosis of GTN is based mainly on the detection of persistent or rising serum βhCG levels, or in the case of PSTT a residual locally invading trophoblastic mass consisting mainly of cytotrophoblasts pathologically. GTN has been prognostically scored using the WHO scoring system and also FIGO anatomic staging (Tables 16.1 and 16.2) [1, 2]. The treatment is based on the WHO score. If the score is ≤ 6, it is considered as low risk and ≥ 7 it is grouped under the high-risk category.

The investigations recommended for proper management are basic complete blood count, serum liver function tests and renal function tests in addition to βhCG. The imaging investigations include a chest radiograph, ultrasonography of the abdomen and the pelvis. CT scan of the lungs may also be done. In patients with pulmonary metastases, a CT scan of the brain is also recommended. Imaging and proper clinical history and examination are mandatory for proper WHO scoring categorisation.

16.1 Low-Risk GTN

The management consists of single-drug treatment with methotrexate/actinomycin D. There are different regimens (Table 16.3) [3].

U. D. Bafna (✉)
Former HOD, Gynaecologic Oncology, Kidwai Memorial Institute of Oncology, Bangalore, India

Department of Gynecologic Oncology, B M Jain Hospital, Bangalore, India

B. Nayak, U. Singh (eds.), *Gestational Trophoblastic Disease*,
https://doi.org/10.1007/978-981-33-4878-3_16

Table 16.1 FIGO staging and classification for gestational trophoblastic neoplasia [1, 2]

FIGO stage	Description
I	Gestational trophoblastic tumours strictly confined to the uterine corpus
II	Gestational trophoblastic tumours extending to the adnexae or to the vagina, but limited to the genital structures
III	Gestational trophoblastic tumours extending to the lungs, with or without genital tract involvement
IV	All other metastatic sites

Table 16.2 WHO scoring system based on prognostic factors [1, 2]

WHO risk factor scoring with FIGO staging	0	1	2	4
Age	<40	>40	–	–
Antecedent pregnancy	Mole	Abortion	Term	
Interval from index pregnancy, months	<4	4–6	7–12	>12
Pretreatment hCG, mIU/mL	$<10^3$	$>10^3$–10^4	$>10^4$–10^5	$>10^5$
Largest tumour size including uterus, cm	–	3–4	≥5	–
Site of metastases including uterus	Lung	Spleen, kidney	Gastrointestinal tract	Brain, liver
Number of metastases identified	–	1–4	5–8	>8
Previous failed chemotherapy	–	–	Single drug	Two or more drugs

Low risk = score 0–6. High risk = ≥7

Table 16.3 First-line single-agent chemotherapy regimens for low-risk gestational trophoblastic neoplasia [3]

- MTX-FA 8-day regimen (50 mg MTX intramuscularly on days 1, 3, 5, 7 with folinic acid 15 mg orally 24 hours after MTX on days 2, 4, 6, 8); repeat every 2 weeks.
- MTX 0.4 mg/kg (max. 25 mg) intravenously or intramuscularly for 5 days every 2 weeks.
- Actinomycin D pulse 1.25 mg/m^2 intravenously every 2 weeks.
- Actinomycin D 0.5 mg intravenously for 5 days every 2 weeks.
- Others: MTX 30–50 mg/m^2 intramuscularly weekly, MTX 300 mg/m^2 infusion every 2 weeks.

Abbreviations: MTX-FA, methotrexate–folinic acid

The most commonly used regimen consists of methotrexate given alternating with folinic acid from day 1 to day 8. The subsequent cycle is repeated on day 15 if there is no clinical toxicity and the blood parameters are within normal range. Usually, 1–2 more cycles of chemotherapy are administered once the βHCG is normalised. About 70–80% respond to first-line methotrexate chemotherapy and the remaining patients respond to either single-agent Actinomycin D or combination chemotherapy which is usually EMA-CO regimen.

It is observed that a risk score of 5–6 and pathological diagnosis of choriocarcinoma has a higher chance of development of resistance to single-agent methotrexate chemotherapy. Methotrexate resistance is diagnosed in the event of rising ß-hCG titres (>10% rise in values of HCG) or plateauing titres (<10% fall or rise in the ß-hCG values at least three values over 3 weeks).

Second-line treatment could be actinomycin D 12 microgram/kg body weight or a fixed dose of 0.5 mg IV on days 1–5. The next cycle is repeated on day 12. Third-line multi-agent combination chemotherapy is considered in non-responders. Surgery for the extirpation of the residual disease in the uterus or elsewhere is rarely required. It is possible to preserve fertility function in almost all cases.

Contraception is advised for a period of 12 months post treatment with chemotherapy. A strict follow-up mainly with regular serum ß-hCG estimations—initially weekly and then fortnightly and then monthly at least for 2 years is mandatory. The menstrual function in the event of chemotherapy-induced amenorrhoea resumes quickly within 2–3 months usually with single-agent chemotherapy treatment.

16.2 High-Risk GTN (WHO Score $\geq$ 7)

High-risk GTN cases are treated with multi-agent chemotherapy. The most commonly used multi-agent chemotherapy is the EMA-CO regimen (etoposide, methotrexate, actinomycin D, cyclophosphamide and vincristine) (Table 16.4) [4]. However, about 20% of patients on EMA-CO therapy develop resistance to the above regimen, but most of such cases can be salvaged with alternative combination therapy. The overall survival rates are as high as 95% in properly treated high-risk patients.

Table 16.4 EMA-CO (etoposide, methotrexate, actinomycin D, cyclophosphamide, vincristine) chemotherapy [4]

Regimens	
Regimen 1	
Day 1	
Etoposide	100 mg/m^2 intravenous infusion over 30 min
Actinomycin D	0.5 mg intravenous bolus
Methotrexate	100 mg/m^2 intravenous bolus 200 mg/m^2 intravenous infusion over 12 h
Day 2	
Etoposide	100 mg/m^2 intravenous infusion over 30 min
Actinomycin D	0.5 mg intravenous bolus
Folinic acid rescue	15 mg intramuscularly or orally every 12 h for four doses (starting 24 h after beginning the methotrexate infusion)
Regimen 2	
Day 8	
Vincristine	1 mg/m^2 intravenous bolus (maximum 2 mg)
Cyclophosphamide	600 mg/m^2 intravenous infusion over 30 min

Table 16.5 Salvage combination chemotherapy [5]

Salvage therapies • EP-EMA (etoposide, cisplatin, etoposide, methotrexate and actinomycin D). • TP/TE (paclitaxel, cisplatin/paclitaxel, etoposide). • MBE (methotrexate, bleomycin, etoposide). • VIP or ICE (etoposide, ifosfamide, and cisplatin or carboplatin). • BEP (bleomycin, etoposide, cisplatin).

16.3 Ultrahigh-Risk Gestational Trophoblastic Neoplasia and Salvage Therapy

The patient with a risk score of ≥13 is grouped under ultrahigh-risk GTN. They carry a poorer prognosis compared to high-risk group as they do present with extensive disease in multiple organs like the brain, liver, lungs, adrenals and kidneys. They are treated initially with low-dose induction chemotherapy followed by standard multi-agent chemotherapy. A good number of such patients develop resistance to conventional regimen and are salvaged with second-line combination chemotherapy (Table 16.5) [5].

The fertility after treatment with combination chemotherapy depends on the number of chemotherapy cycles. More than 5–6 cycles of combination chemotherapy may result in decreased ovarian reserve and premature ovarian failure resulting in prolonged secondary amenorrhea and premature onset of menopause. In these patients who usually have a higher WHO score of ≥13, there is hardly any time for oocyte retrieval and preservation before the administration of chemotherapy as the tumour doubling time is very short. The use of GnRH analogues to suppress ovarian function during chemotherapy to minimise chemotherapy-induced damage of the ovarian antral follicles is controversial with not much published data [6]. However, the pregnancy rate after single-agent and multi-agent chemotherapy is comparable to that of the general population. Moreover, there was no difference in the risk of miscarriage, ectopic pregnancy, repeat molar pregnancy and stillbirth in comparison to the general population [7].

16.4 Role of Fertility Sparing Surgery

Some patients with high-risk GTT may present with uterine perforation due to the tumour. In some of these patients, a conservative surgery to debulk the uterine tumour may be considered as the residual tumour can rapidly respond to the postoperative definitive chemotherapy. This may amount to a segmental resection or repair. Such surgery has to be done with utmost care as the tissues are friable and lead to brisk haemorrhage. Risk of rupture in future pregnancies have to be counselled. Evacuation of residual mole may sometimes prove beneficial and can be done under ultrasonographic guidance to preserve the uterus, decrease risk of perforation and reduce the cycles of chemotherapy. Ultrasound guided intratumoural injection of methotrexate has been tried with encouraging results. This is an alternative option in single agent resistant focus to avoid multiagent chemotherapy [8].

In chemoresistant GTT, with uterine residual resistant focus of the tumour, similarly, a conservative resection of the tumour may be considered preserving the uterus for fertility [9].

Follow-Up: Contraception is advised for a period of 12 months post treatment with chemotherapy. A strict follow-up mainly with regular serum b HCG estimations—initially weekly and then fortnightly and then monthly at least for 2 years is mandatory.

16.5 PSTT/ETT

Both PSTT and ETT are relatively chemoresistant. They are best treated by hysterectomy. When fertility is an issue, segmental excision with or without lymphadenectomy can be offered in localised lesions.

References

1. FIGO Committee on Gynecologic Oncology. Current FIGO staging for cancer of the vagina, fallopian tube, ovary, and gestational trophoblastic neoplasia. Int J Gynecol Obstet. 2009;105(1):3–4.
2. Ngan H, Bender H, Benedet JL, Jones H, Montruccoli GC, Pecorelli S, FIGO Committee on Gynecologic Oncology. Gestational trophoblastic neoplasia, FIGO 2000 staging and classification. Int J Gynaecol Obstet. 2003;83(Suppl 1):175–7.
3. Lawrie TA, Alazzam M, Tidy J, Hancock BW, Osborne R. First-line chemotherapy in low-risk gestational trophoblastic neoplasia. Cochrane Database Syst Rev. 2016;
4. Deng L, Zhang J, Wu T. Combination chemotherapy for primary treatment of high risk gestational trophoblastic tumour. Cochrane Database Syst Rev. 2003;
5. Lurain JR, Schink JC. Importance of salvage therapy in the management of high-risk gestational trophoblastic neoplasia. J Reprod Med. 2012;57:219–24.
6. Abdel-Razeq H. Gonadotropin-releasing hormone agonists during chemotherapy for ovarian function and fertility preservation for patients with early-stage breast cancer. Cancer Manag Res. 2019;11:4273–82.
7. Williams J, Short D, Dayal L, Strickland S, Harvey R, Tin T, et al. Effect of early pregnancy following chemotherapy on disease relapse and fetal outcome in women treated for gestational trophoblastic neoplasia. J Reprod Med. 2014;59(5–6):248–54.
8. Tsukihara S, et al. Ultrasound-guided local injection of methotrexate to treat an invasive hydatidiform mole. 2004;30(3):202–4.
9. Bafna UD, Ahuja VK, Umadevi K, et al. Gestational trophoblastic tumours-situation analysis in a third world regional cancer centre. Int J Gyn Cancer. 1997;7:197–204.

Follow-Up of Gestational Trophoblastic Disease: How Often and How Long

17

Jaydip Bhaumik and S. K. Giri

This has already been discussed in previous chapters that gestational trophoblastic disease (GTD) is a group of conditions showing abnormal proliferation of the trophoblast. At one end of the spectrum of the disease is partial or complete molar pregnancy that, on a majority of instances, behaves like a benign condition but has the potential to recur and metastasise like a malignant lesion. At the other extreme, there is the more aggressive malignant disease of choriocarcinoma. Follow-up strategies are therefore tailored according to the correct diagnosis and treatment given if any.

In a population-based study in the Netherlands [1], among the registered hydatidiform mole patients (N-365), 75% attained spontaneous normalisation following evacuation of the molar pregnancy, and only one patient (0.38%) out of them subsequently required chemotherapy due to rising titre of ßhCG after 8 weeks of normalisation. They also quoted that two normal values of ßhCG after treatment of complete mole are enough to remove patients from surveillance. Relapse rates among those who needed chemotherapy treatment were 8.1 and 6.3% for the low and high-risk category, respectively. It was evident that although rare, the possibility of recurrence was still there even after normalisation of ßhCG values among patients who did not receive chemotherapy as their treatment for molar pregnancy. However, if they needed chemotherapy, the risk of recurrence remained significant, irrespective of their being low risk or high risk and hence warrant stringent follow-up.

The current chapter addresses the dilemma and justification of an effective strategy for monitoring women with GTD in an Indian setting and to define how often and how long they should be kept under surveillance.

J. Bhaumik (✉)
Gynaecological Oncology, Tata Medical Center, Kolkata, India
e-mail: Jaydip.bhaumik@tmckolkata.com

S. K. Giri
PG Department of Gynaecologic Oncology, A.H. Post Graduate Institute of Cancer, Cuttack, India

B. Nayak, U. Singh (eds.), *Gestational Trophoblastic Disease*,
https://doi.org/10.1007/978-981-33-4878-3_17

17.1 Whom to Monitor

All women diagnosed with GTD need monitoring.

A partial mole may be an incidental diagnosis on histological examination of the retained products of conception after a miscarriage. Hence, it is advisable to subject all surgically evacuated specimens for histological examination. If pathological review is unavailable, human chorionic gonadotrophin should be measured three to four weeks after the termination of pregnancy to identify women with persistently raised values who need to be followed up [2]. Routine pathological examination of products of conception after the termination of a viable pregnancy is not recommended. The risk of a coincidental molar pregnancy with viable pregnancy is low; estimated to be 1 in 20,000 [3].

The incidence of molar pregnancy among women with incomplete miscarriage may vary from population to population. A hospital-based study from Tanzania reported an incidence of 12.8% of molar pregnancy among women undergoing surgical evacuation after diagnosis of incomplete miscarriage. This was more common among women younger than 20 years of age [4].

Molar pregnancy, especially a partial mole may be missed on a previous ultrasound scan that confirmed early fetal demise or an incomplete miscarriage. It is also important that the pathologist examining the tissues of products of conception is experienced to differentiate between molar degeneration of trophoblastic tissue and a true hydatidiform mole. The majority of these women after evacuation of the mole will have their ßhCG declining at a steady pace and eventually become undetectable in less than 10 weeks [5].

Patients with complete hydatidiform mole (CHM) in whom ßhCG value normalises by 56th day have less chance of developing persistent disease as compared to those who take a longer time to fall, in whom there is a 3.8-fold higher risk of developing GTN [6]. Hence, women belonging to the earlier group require a short follow-up of 6 months from the date of evacuation against a longer follow-up of 6 months from the date of normalisation of ßhCG in the latter group [7]. In partial hydatidiform mole (PHM), the risk of persistence is extremely low; hence, one normal ßhCG value one month after ßhCG normalisation is sufficient [6].

There is another group of women in whom ßhCG plateaus or shows rising titre during follow up; they are termed as gestational trophoblastic neoplasia (GTN). They require chemotherapy, single or multiple regimens, depending on the stage and WHO score with regular follow-up.

There is yet another group of GTN, who are diagnosed with Choriocarcinoma (CCA) at the outset. A study from Peking Union Medical College Hospital reported a recurrence rate of 4.3% of 490 women treated for CCA [8]. The same group also reported a better outcome for the patients who relapsed compared to those who were chemoresistant [9]. This study reiterated the importance of follow-up of patients with CCA who showed complete remission after initial chemotherapy.

17.2 How Long to Follow Up

There is no consensus of opinion regarding how long these women be monitored. Different protocols from different authors are as follows:

ESMO practical guideline advocates lifelong monitoring after chemotherapy, as recurrence may be delayed by several years [10]. In the UK, the follow-up protocol with ßhCG after complete remission of GTN is elaborate: ßhCG is monitored weekly for 6 weeks after chemotherapy (CT), then every fortnight for 6 months, monthly thereafter for 1 to 2 years, then 6 monthly for 5 years [10].

In one more population-based study from 1958 to 2015, of 4000 cases of treated GTN, low and high risk, Balachandran *et al.* did not find any recurrences after 7 years of follow-up; hence, they recommended a surveillance of 10 years instead of a lifetime follow-up [11].

However, the above protocol may not be feasible for many other countries. It should be the discretion of the physician and the affordability of the patient, based on which the follow-up protocol should be devised for each individual patient.

One of the most recent articles recommends that all patients of low-risk GTN who have been treated with single-agent CT be treated with 2–3 more cycles of CT after normalisation of ßhCG and followed up with monthly ßhCG for 6 months. Patients with high-risk GTN with multi-agent CT will require 3 or 4 cycles of CT after normalisation of ßhCG followed by monthly monitoring for 12 months and 6 monthly for 5 years. Pregnancy may be allowed after completion of 6 months' follow-up in low-risk group and 1 year of follow-up in the high-risk group [12].

Hence, taking different viewpoints into account, follow-up for both low-risk and high-risk GTN cases should be at least for one year, and pregnancy be allowed after one year of follow-up. However, in high-risk cases, follow-up should be stringent at least for 24 months, maybe lifetime, although the chance of recurrence after one year in those groups of patients is minimal [13].

17.3 How to Monitor

WHO recommends that all women diagnosed with GTD are monitored with weekly ßhCG until on three consecutive occasions the values remain undetectable [4]. There is no consensus of opinion regarding how long will these women be monitored.

The mode of follow-up will also depend on the availability of resources. These women who are diagnosed with hydatidiform mole are young and are likely to plan for pregnancy after recovering from the initial disease episode. Also, the risk of recurrence is highest in the first year. It may therefore be justified to continue monitoring the ßhCG levels at regular intervals (depending on the available resources) after it has come back to normal values for at least 6 months to one year depending on the situation, during which time the woman should be instructed to use contraception to avoid pregnancy. Combined oral contraceptives are the best contraceptive used as soon as ßhCG normalises. Rarely relapse may occur in women who had successful pregnancies subsequent to a molar pregnancy [14]. Many institutions will therefore prefer to monitor for many years even after subsequent pregnancies. In all future pregnancies, pathologic examination of the placenta or other products of conception as well as determination of a 6-week postpartum ßhCG level are recommended.

17.4 Summary of Follow-Up Schedule of GTD

PHM

– Stop follow-up after one normal ßhCG value 1 month after ßhCG normalisation.

CHM

– If normal fall within 56th day—follow up for 6 months after evacuation.
– If fall is delayed beyond 56th day—follow up for 6 months after normalisation of ßhCG.

GTN- Criteria

1. Plateau of ßhCG lasts for 4 measurements over a period of 3 weeks or longer, i.e. days 1, 7, 14, 21 (plateau is usually defined as variation of values ±10%).
2. Rise of tumour ßhCG on three consecutive weekly measurements, over a period of 2 weeks or longer, days 1, 7, 14 (usually defined as an increase of >10%).
3. Histological diagnosis of CCA.

Follow-up schedule of GTN: based on various European and north American guidelines. (Note: Charing Cross Hospital, London follows-up indefinitely.) [15].

- Low-risk GTN: (post Methotrexate/actinomycin): Follow up with monthly ßhCG for 12 months.
- High-risk GTN: (post EMA-CO or equivalent): Follow up with monthly ßhCG for 2 years.
- PSTT/ETT: Follow up for a minimum of 5 years—ßhCG plus appropriate imaging.

It must be emphasised that the primary aim of the follow-up policy is for early detection of relapses to improve survival. GTDs are potentially curable conditions, and therefore, all efforts should be made to keep the woman under close surveillance at reasonable intervals for a reasonable duration of time.

Protocol for Serial hCG Measurements—After Surgical Treatment of Hydatidiform Mole

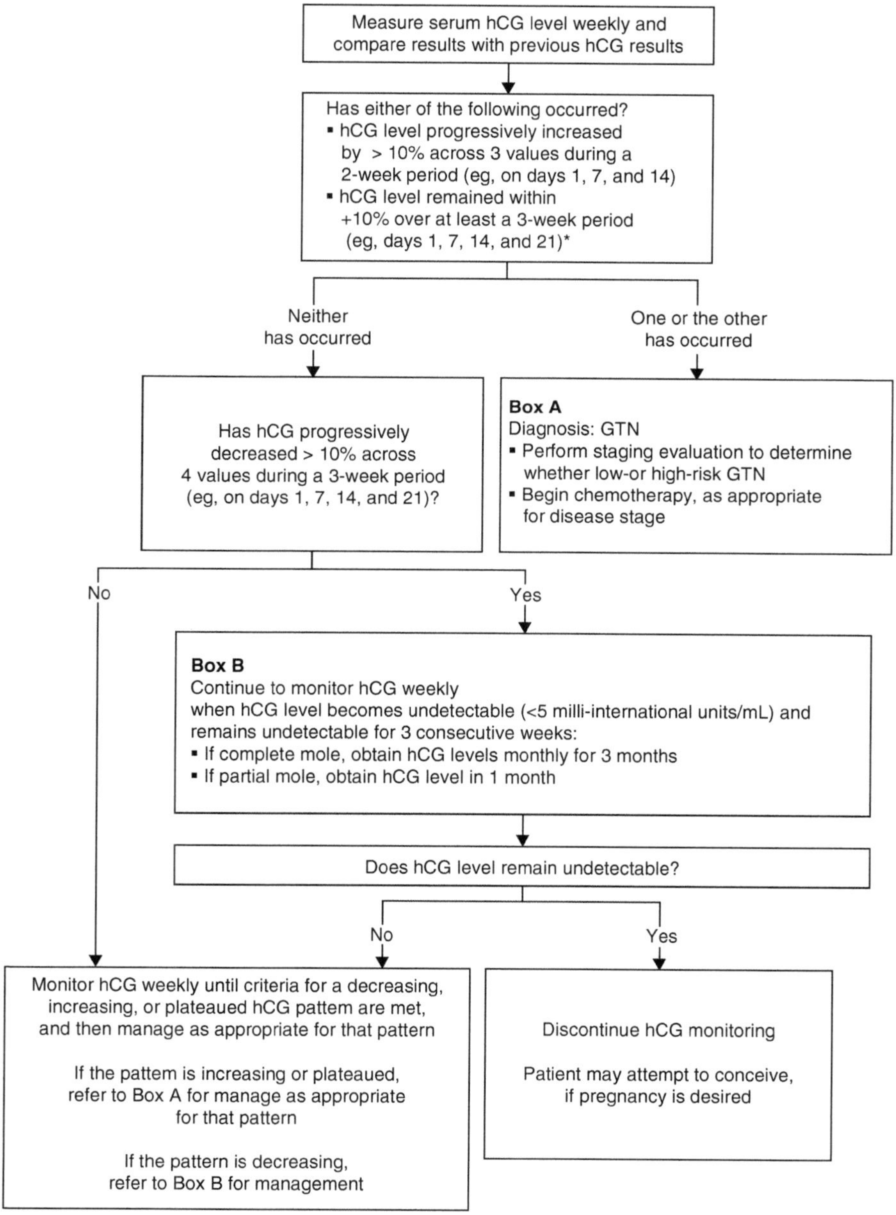

Hydatidiform mole: Treatment and follow-up—Up to Date, Jan 2020.

References

1. Kerkmeijer L, Wielsma S, Massuger L, Sweep F, Thomas C. Recurrent gestational trophoblastic disease after hCG normalization following hydatidiform mole in The Netherlands. Gynecol Oncol. 2007;106:142–6. https://doi.org/10.1016/j.ygyno.2007.03.010.
2. Seckl MJ, Gillmore R, Foskett M, Sebire NJ, Rees H, Newlands ES. Routine terminations of pregnancy—shouldwe screenfor gestational trophoblastic neoplasia? Lancet. 2004;364:705–7.
3. Seckl MJ, Gillmore R, Foskett MA, Sebire NJ, Rees H, Newlands ES. Routine terminations of pregnancies: should we screen for gestational trophoblastic neoplasia? Lancet. 2004;364:705–7.
4. Kitange B, Matovelo D, Konje E, Massinde A, Rambau P. Hydatidiform moles among patients with incomplete abortion in Mwanza City, North western Tanzania. Afr Health Sci. 2015 Dec;15(4):1081–6.
5. https://www.who.int/selection_medicines/committees/expert/20/applications/GestationalTrophobla sticNeoplasia.pdf
6. Coyle C, Short D, Jackson L, et al. What is optimal duration of human chorionic gonadotrophin surveillance following evacuation of a molar pregnancy? A retrospective analysis on over 20,000 consecutive patients. Gynecol Oncol. 2008;148:254–7.
7. The management of gestational trophoblastic disease. Green–top Guideline No. 38 February 2010.
8. Sun Y, Xiang Y, Wan XR, Yang XY. Factors related to recurrence of choriocarcinoma and evaluation of treatment outcomes (article in Chinese). Zhonghua Fu Chan KeZaZhi. 2006;41(5):329–32.
9. Feng F, Xiang Y, Wan X, Zhou Y. Prognosis of patients with relapsed and chemoresistant gestational trophoblastic neoplasia transferred to the Peking union medical college hospital. BJOG. 2010;117(1):47–52.
10. Seckl MJ, Sebire NJ, Fisher RA, Golfier F, Massuger L, Sessa C, on behalf of the ESMO Guidelines Working Group. Gestational trophoblastic disease: ESMO clinical practice guidelines for diagnosis, treatment and follow-up. Ann Oncol. 2013;24(Suppl 6):vi39–50.
11. Balachandran K, Salawu A, Ghorani E, Kaur B, Sebire NJ, Short D, Harvey R, Hancock B, Tidy J, Singh K, Sarwar N, Winter MC, Seckl MJ. When to stop human chorionic gonadotrophin (hCG) surveillance after treatment with chemotherapy for gestational trophoblastic neoplasia (GTN): a national analysis on over 4,000 patients. Gynecol Oncol. 2019;155(1):8. Epub 2019 Jul 30
12. Braga A, Mora P, de Melo AC, Rodrigues AN, Junior JA, Filho JR, Seckl MJ. Challenges in the diagnosis and treatment of gestational trophoblastic neoplasia worldwide. World J Clin Oncol. 2019;10(2):28–37.
13. Goldstein DP, Berkowitz RS, Horowitz NS. Presentation and management of gestational trophoblastic neoplasia in the USA. In: Hancock BW, Seckl MJ, Berkowitz RS, editors. Gestational trophoblastic disease. 4th ed. ISSTD:2015.
14. Seckl MJ, Fisher RA, Salerno G, Rees H, Paradinas FJ, Foskett MA, Newlands ES. Choriocarcinoma and partial hydatidiform moles. Lancet. 2000;356:36–9.
15. New Zealand Gynaecologic Cancer Group Guidelines, 3. 12. 2018.

Establishment of Regional Centers for Gestational Trophoblastic Disease Follow-Up and Referral and Gestational Trophoblastic Disease Registry

18

Professor Sekharan Paradan K

18.1 Introduction

Gestational Trophoblastic Disease (GTD) develops as a result of abnormal proliferation of placental trophoblast and includes the benign complete and partial hydatidiform moles (CHM and PHM) as well as the malignant versions such as Choriocarcinoma (CC), invasive mole (IM), Placental Site Trophoblastic Tumor (PSTT), and Epithelioid Trophoblastic Tumor (ETT). The malignant forms of the condition are collectively referred to as Gestational Trophoblastic Neoplasia (GTN).

Regular surveillance following hydatidiform mole is crucial for the timely detection and management of the potentially fatal gestational trophoblastic neoplasia. Such fatalities are avoidable if there is a system of regular follow-up using highly sensitive and validated hCG assay platforms. Regional GTD referral centers play a key role in ensuring optimum diagnosis and management of Gestational Trophoblastic Neoplasia.

GTD centers should have a standardized evidence-based protocol to diagnose and manage cases of gestational trophoblastic disease and in addition foster research by facilitating prospective studies. Clinical datasets should be stored in a secure electronic format and made accessible for future analyses.

18.2 The Setting

GTD referral centers and the associated registries can be started in Government/Private teaching hospitals with the aim of developing a network of expertise including the departments of Obstetrics and Gynecology, Gynecologic oncology, Medical,

S. Paradan K (✉)
Department of Obstetrics and Gynaecology, Government Medical College, Calicut, India

Formerly working at Government Medical College, Calicut, India

B. Nayak, U. Singh (eds.), *Gestational Trophoblastic Disease*,
https://doi.org/10.1007/978-981-33-4878-3_18

Surgical and Radiation oncology, clinical imaging facilities (including ultrasonography [USG], CT, and MRI scanning), pathologists with expertise in the diagnosis of GTD and a clinical chemistry laboratory service with facilities for hormonal assays. These centers should set up outpatient GTD referral clinics on fixed days of the week with standardized pathways accessible to all referring physicians that should stipulate the minimum dataset required to make a referral to GTD centers. Oversight and supervision will be the responsibility of a group of clinicians who wish to develop a special interest in GTD within the department of Obstetrics and Gynecology and led by senior faculty members with expertise in GTD management. All referred cases should be streamlined for registration and review in this clinic. The services should include counseling and psychological support for the patient and her family. Funding for such GTD centers may be collaboratively secured from state and central government departments as well as charitable organizations. GTD centers should register, monitor, and treat women with gestational trophoblastic disease as well as audit treatment outcomes and maintain prospective clinical datasets for education and research. They should also host a website that provides relevant information to referring physicians and patients. A network of communication including appropriate use of electronic and social media should be set up to foster long-term relationships between GTD centers, referring physicians, and patients.

18.3 The Registry

The protocol-based prospective analysis and treatment results of GTD cases should be recorded and maintained in electronic format for future research and evaluation of treatment results. This should also allow effective communication with patients to ensure engagement with their care, monitoring, and education. Treatment results of various regimens should be collated with details of USG findings, β-hCG values, and histopathological results along with epidemiological data (Data collection sheet is attached as Appendix).

18.4 The Key Ingredients

1. Diagnosis of molar pregnancy
2. Sensitive hCG assay
3. The expert clinical team
4. Protocol-based management

18.5 Diagnosis: Ultrasonography and Histopathological Evaluation

The classical presentation of a molar pregnancy with uterine size disproportionately larger than the period of amenorrhea, associated with hyperemesis, bleeding, bilateral lutein cysts, early-onset preeclampsia, and thyrotoxicosis is rare nowadays, thanks to the availability of USG in the early evaluation of pregnancy [1]. Molar changes may be evident on ultrasonography beyond 10 weeks, and pathological confirmation is usually straightforward in the late first trimester or in the early second trimester. However, it may be difficult to make a diagnosis of hydatidiform mole if a USG is performed for vaginal bleeding in early pregnancy at ≤8 weeks and reported as a failing pregnancy. Hence, all products of conception should be sent for histopathological evaluation in such instances. The services of an expert pathologist are essential for the diagnosis of molar pregnancy in the first trimester. Facilities for immunohistochemistry for imprinted genes such as $p57^{kip2}$ [2] may be necessary in certain cases. The timely diagnosis of a molar pregnancy is crucial for such patients to be registered for regular follow-up. Further clarification of the diagnosis as complete or partial mole is also important given the differences in the risk of malignant transformation (15–20% in complete mole versus 1–5% in partial mole).

18.6 Expert Pathologist

The classical pathological appearance of late first trimester or early second-trimester hydatidiform mole may not be present in early first trimester hydatidiform mole, and therefore, the input of an expert pathologist is necessary to establish the diagnosis. Development of GTN is not dependent on gestational age at evacuation but on the type of abnormal pregnancy, i.e., complete versus partial mole [3]. Such differentiation is a key step in ensuring regular follow-up for the patient group at high risk of GTN.

18.7 hCG Assay

Human Chorionic Gonadotrophin (hCG) is a highly sensitive tumor marker for the follow-up and management of GTD. All types of trophoblastic cells secrete hCG; however, in GTN, there is a higher incidence of abnormal hCG molecules compared to normal pregnancy. Routine hCG assay systems used for the confirmation of pregnancy may not pick up abnormal types of hCG seen in GTN. Assay platforms that reliably detect and quantify all types of hCG, including hyperglycosylated hCG, nicked hCG, free β-hCG, and hCG without C-terminal should be used in GTD centers for surveillance of GTD patients. The Siemens IMMULITE system has been validated for accurate detection of such abnormal hCG types seen in malignant trophoblastic disease [4]. Whenever the hCG level does not correlate with the clinical scenario, alternative assays should be used to rule out false-positive results. Phantom hCG due to heterophilic antibodies can be excluded by testing for the presence of hCG in the urine which will be absent in cases of spurious assay results.

18.8 The Clinical Team

The head of the department of Obstetrics and Gynecology should have operational oversight of GTD centers. The department should run a specialist clinic, "The Trophoblastic Disease Clinic" on a fixed day of the week, separate from the routine OP day of the unit. A senior member of the faculty, preferably from the unit of the head of the department, will be responsible for running the clinic. They will be assisted by other junior faculty members and postgraduate students. All patients will be registered in the GTD center and prospectively followed up according to the standard operating protocol. The patients diagnosed with Gestational Trophoblastic Neoplasia (GTN) should be assessed by the tumor board to decide on the indications for chemotherapy and the particular regimen for each patient.

18.9 The Tumor Board

The board will be chaired by the head of the department of obstetrics and gynecology and consist of the faculty member in charge of the GTD clinic, gynecological oncologist, medical oncologist, surgical oncologist, radiation oncologist, and the pathologist. The board should schedule regular meetings at least on a fortnightly basis to recommend individualized management plans for patients including the appropriate chemotherapeutic regimen.

18.10 Ultrasonography

The classic ultrasonographic appearance of "snowstorm" appearance of CHM is rarely seen nowadays as ultrasonography is performed early for evaluation of pregnancy [5] especially if they present with bleeding or other symptoms in the first trimester. Suspicious cases should undergo evacuation under general anesthesia after preliminary evaluation and the products should be submitted for histopathological examination by the expert pathologist. The typical histopathological features will not be evident in the early stages (≤8 weeks), and therefore, this requires input from such experts.

Early-stage molar pregnancy may be misdiagnosed as anembryonic pregnancy, blighted ovum, or missed abortion and managed by medical abortion. Such patients may expel the products of conception at home, and it is likely that no histopathological examination will be made. Therefore, all products of conception in early pregnancy loss should be submitted for histopathological analysis even if USG does not suggest typical molar pregnancy [6, 7]. Early evacuation of a molar pregnancy alone does not reduce the risk of subsequent development of GTN. It is advisable to perform a urine pregnancy test 4 weeks after any abortion to confirm regression of hCG levels to baseline. Any persistent elevation in hCG levels at this stage warrants further evaluation.

18.11 Registration

All patients with a diagnosis of Gestational Trophoblastic Disease should be registered in the specialist referral centers. Patients should sign a form after informed consent confirming their willingness to have the necessary follow-up as per the management protocol including the relevant investigations and treatment and consent for the use of their anonymized clinical data for research purposes. Patients should be assigned a unique ID for the retrieval of their data. Contact details should be stored separately to encourage adherence to follow-up visits.

18.12 The Protocol

All patients with suspected molar pregnancy should undergo suction evacuation under general anesthesia, preferably with ultrasound guidance. Pre-evacuation hCG assay and complete blood count are mandatory. With a larger uterine size and a higher risk of heavy bleeding, oxytocin infusion may be considered to reduce the bleeding during evacuation. Gentle curettage of the uterine cavity will help to ensure complete evacuation. The specimen should be submitted for histopathological examination to confirm the diagnosis and type of molar pregnancy—especially to differentiate complete from partial hydatidiform mole. Rh-negative patients should receive anti-D immunoglobulin. Following evacuation, patients are advised to use low-dose COC pills for contraception.

Patients are then asked to report 1 week after evacuation for ultrasonographic evaluation to ensure complete evacuation of the products of conception. Repeat curettage is not indicated if there is no USG evidence of retained tissue.

18.13 Prophylactic Chemotherapy

Routine use of prophylactic chemotherapy at the time of the evacuation of the mole is not recommended. Patients with high-risk features such as uterine size 4 weeks more than period of amenorrhea, pre-evacuation hCG of 100,000 IU/L and above, bilateral theca lutein cysts, elderly multiparas, and those who may not have reliable follow-up may benefit from prophylactic chemotherapy. A proportion of these patients may develop GTN and have resistant disease.

18.14 Follow-Up

All patients after evacuation of a molar pregnancy should have regular follow-up with weekly serum β-hCG assay until negative, to enable early diagnosis of GTN and ensure complete cure.

In complete mole, if β-hCG becomes negative within 8 weeks of evacuation, only six more months' follow-up is required from the date of evacuation. If more than 8 weeks are required for β-hCG to normalize, then six additional months' follow-up is required from the date of normalization of hCG with monthly β-hCG measurements. In cases of partial hydatidiform mole, following hCG normalization, a repeat hCG evaluation is done after 1 month and if negative, no further follow-up is required [8, 9].

18.15 Diagnosis of GTN

- Rising trend (>10% increase) in hCG across three values over two consecutive weeks
- Plateauing of four consecutive values over 3 weeks (<10% fall from the previous week)
- Persistence of hCG more than 6 months following evacuation
- Histological diagnosis of choriocarcinoma

Once the diagnosis of GTN is made, the patient is managed by the gynecologic oncology/medical oncology team. In our institution (Government Medical College, Calicut, Kerala), low-risk cases requiring single-agent chemotherapy are managed by the gynecology team running the follow-up clinics with expert input from the tumor board.

18.16 Evaluation of Metastases in GTN

Once the diagnosis of GTN is confirmed, further imaging must be arranged to detect metastases and for staging and risk scoring. Chest X-ray may be adequate for the detection of lung metastasis. Pelvic ultrasonography with Doppler study will help to identify localized growth in the uterus. If chest X-ray confirms secondaries, then CT abdomen and MRI brain should also be performed [10].

18.17 Staging and Risk Score to Determine Choice of Chemotherapy

FIGO 2000 Anatomical staging and the modified WHO scoring adopted by FIGO in 2000 [11] are used worldwide to determine the type of chemotherapy and is recommended for risk stratification.

GTN with FIGO stage I, II, and III and a risk score of ≤6 are treated with single-agent chemotherapy.

GTN with FIGO stage I, II, and III risk with a risk score of ≥7 or stage IV are treated with multi-agent chemotherapy.

18.18 Choice of Single-Agent Chemotherapy for Low-Risk GTN

Based on our experience [12] of achieving 92.9% cure with a Methotrexate and Folinic rescue regimen (MTX/FA) in the management low-risk GTN, this is the treatment of choice in low-risk patients.

18.18.1 MTX/FA Rescue Regimen

Inj. methotrexate 1 mg/kg on days 1, 3, 5, and 7 and inj. Folinic acid on days 2, 4, 6, and 8 by intramuscular route. Folinic acid is given 24 h after methotrexate. The course is repeated every 2 weeks and two to three additional courses are recommended after hCG assays become negative. Complete blood count, LFT, and RFT are done before starting every course. Anemia, infection, and impaired liver and renal function will aggravate the toxicity of methotrexate.

18.18.2 Actinomycin-D

Actinomycin-D is an effective single agent for low-risk GTN, and the usual regimen is 0.5 mg I/V for 5 days, repeated every 2 weeks. Extravasation of Actinomycin will result in sloughing of the local area with severe pain (local infiltration with 100 mg Hydrocortisone and 2 ml of 1% Xylocaine will reduce the severity of such local reaction).

18.19 Low-Risk GTN with Score 5 and 6

It is reported that low-risk GTN with scores of 5 and 6 may not respond well to single-agent chemotherapy. In order to reduce the toxicity, such patients may also be treated using single-agent chemotherapy and the majority may respond. For those who are showing poor response with hCG levels between 100 and 300 IU/L, a second agent such as Actinomycin-D following MTX/FA regimen may achieve cure. The patients with a risk score of 5 and 6 showing poor response to a single agent with hCG levels above 300 IU/L will require multi-agent therapy.

18.20 High-Risk GTN

High-risk GTN is managed by EMA-CO regimen (etoposide, methotrexate, actinomycin-D, cyclophosphamide, and vincristine). Patients who fail to respond to EMA-CO can be managed with salvage therapies such as EP-EMA, TP/TE, MBE, ICE, or BEP regimens achieving a cure rate of 95%.

18.21 Ultrahigh-Risk GTN

Patients with a risk score of 13 and above and with massive liver and brain metastases do poorly when treated with first-line multi-agent chemotherapy. Standard chemotherapy may cause sudden tumor collapse with bleeding, metabolic acidosis, myelosuppression, septicemia, and multiorgan failure which may be fatal. They are best managed by induction therapy with etoposide 100 mg/m^2 and Cisplatin 20 mg/m^2 on days 1 and 2, repeated weekly for 1–3 weeks before starting the full regimen.

18.22 Follow-Up After GTN

After treatment of GTN, follow-up with monthly hCG assays is required for 1 year for identification of relapses. Patients should be advised of reliable contraception during follow-up. Future fertility, pregnancy, and babies are not affected. Patients who had molar pregnancy without development of GTN need not have any follow-up after subsequent pregnancy.

18.23 Twin Pregnancy with Mole and Baby

There is no extra risk of malignancy in twins with normal fetus and pregnancy may be allowed to continue after counseling regarding the risk of bleeding and need for surgical management, after confirming the normality of the baby by amniocentesis and karyotyping.

18.24 Role of Surgery

Emergency laparotomy and hysterectomy may be required in cases of invasive mole leading to perforation of uterus with severe intraperitoneal bleeding. Neurosurgery may be required in cases of intracranial bleeding or raised intracranial pressure. Resection of localized drug-resistant tumor may also be curative.

18.25 Our Experience

The author's group has started a trophoblastic disease follow-up and referral center at Government Medical College, Calicut, Kerala, in 1990. Calicut Medical College serves as the tertiary care teaching hospital catering to the four northern districts of Kerala with an annual delivery rate of more than 25,000 deliveries during this period. From 1990 to 2005, we had 1569 cases of hydatidiform mole, and 321 cases were diagnosed as GTN (20.4%). By ensuring regular follow-up of cases, GTN was diagnosed at a very early stage and 92.9% had complete cure with Methotrexate and Folinic Acid. Patients needing single-agent chemotherapy were treated in the Gynecology department. Only 7.1% needed multi-agent chemotherapy [12]. There were no fatalities and many patients subsequently conceived and had normal deliveries. The center continues to function well as a leading center for trophoblastic diseases.

Appendix

Data collection for GTD register
  Name —————— Age ——————
  Address ——————
  Mail ID —————— Phone no. ——————
  Parity—————— LMP ——————
  Period of gestation in weeks ——————
  Clinical presentation
  Hyperemesis —————— Bleeding P/V ——————
Passing of vesicles ——————
  USG findings ——————
Complete mole/partial mole ——————
  Blood gp. CBC, TSH, Pre-evacuation hCG
  Method of evacuation ——————
  Histopathology
  USG after 1 week- residual products- repeat curettage.
Weekly serum hCG hCG after 4 weeks (> 20,000 IU/L—Chemotherapy)
  Post evacuation bleeding
Persistence of lutein cysts Sub-urethral nodule
Plateauing/rise in hCG GTN
Metastatic workup X-ray chest, USG abdomen, CT abdomen, MRI brain
  Chemotherapy regimen
  No. of courses—Response
  Follow-up

References

1. P K Sekharan, Gestational trophoblastic disease, review article. J Obstet Gynecol. 2008; 58(4):299–307.
2. Sebire NJ. The diagnosis of gestational trophoblastic disease in early pregnancy: implications for screening, counseling and management. Ultrasound Obstet Gynecol. 2005;25:421–4.
3. Seckl MJ, Dhillon T, Dancey G, Foskett M, Paradinas FJ, Rees HC, Sebire NJ, Vigushin DM, Newlands ES. Increased gestational age at evacuation of a complete hydatidiform mole: does it correlate with increased risk of requiring chemotherapy? J Reprod Med. 2004;49:527–30.
4. Laurence A. Cole, hCG, the wonder of today's science. Reprod Biol Endocrinol. 2012;10:24.
5. Mangili G, Lorusso D, Brown J, Pfisterer J, Massuger L, Vaughan M, Ngan HYS, Golfier F, Sekharan PK, Charry RC, Poveda A, Kim J-W, Xiang Y, Berkowtiz R, Seckl MJ. Trophoblastic disease review for diagnosis and management, a joint report from the International Society for

the Study of trophoblastic disease, European organisation for the treatment of trophoblastic disease, and the gynecologic cancer inter group. Int J Gynecol Cancer. 2014;24:S109YS116.
6. The Management of Gestational Trophoblastic Disease Green–top Guideline No. 38, February 2010.
7. Management of Gestational Trophoblastic Disease, Green-top Guideline No. 38, 3 Peer Review Draft–January 2019.
8. Ngan HYS, Seckl MJ, Berkowitz RS, Xiang Y, Golfiere F, Sekharan PK, Lurain JR. Update on the diagnosis and management of gestational trophoblastic disease-Figo cancer report. Int J Gynecol Obstet. 2015;131(2015):S123–6.
9. Ngan HYS, Seckl MJ, Berkowitz RS, Yang X, Golfier F, Sekharan PK, Lurain JR, Massuger L, Figo Cancer Report. Update on the diagnosis and management of gestational, trophoblastic disease. Int J Gynecol Obstet. 2018;143(Suppl. 2):79–85.
10. Seckl MJ, Sebire NJ, Fisher RA, Golfier F, Massuger L, Sessa C. Gestational trophoblastic disease: ESMO clinical practice guidelines for diagnosis, treatment and follow-up. Ann Oncol. 2013;24(Suppl 6):vi39–50. doi:10.1093/annonc/mdt345 Published online 1 September 2013
11. FIGO Oncology Committee. FIGO staging for gestational trophoblastic neoplasia 2000. Int J Gynaecol Obstet. 2002;77(3):285–7.
12. Sekharan PK, Sreedevi NS, Radhadevi VP, Rasheeda BO, Raghavan J, Guhan B. Management of postmolar gestational trophoblastic disease with methotrexate and folinic acid: 15 years of experience. J Reprod Med. 2006;51:835–40.

Correction to: Human Chorionic Gonadotropin

Ashok Kumar Padhy, Deepika Dash, and Richi Khandelwal

Correction to:
B. Nayak, U. Singh (eds.), Gestational Trophoblastic Disease, https://doi.org/10.1007/978-981-33-4878-3_4

The book was inadvertently published with an incorrect spelling of the author's first name in Chapter 4 as "Rich" whereas it should be "Richi". This error has now been corrected with this erratum.

The updated online version of this chapter can be found at
https://doi.org/10.1007/978-981-33-4878-3_4

B. Nayak, U. Singh (eds.), *Gestational Trophoblastic Disease*,
https://doi.org/10.1007/978-981-33-4878-3_19

GPSR Compliance

The European Union's (EU) General Product Safety Regulation (GPSR) is a set of rules that requires consumer products to be safe and our obligations to ensure this.

If you have any concerns about our products, you can contact us on ProductSafety@springernature.com

In case Publisher is established outside the EU, the EU authorized representative is:

Springer Nature Customer Service Center GmbH
Europaplatz 3
69115 Heidelberg, Germany

Batch number: 10732044

Printed by Printforce, the Netherlands